Behold the man!

He stands idle, his back turned to the beauty
of the foaming sea.

He stares, uncomprehending, at the
sand beneath his boots.

His mind, clouded and dark as the tumultuous
sky above, churns like the storm-riled sea.

His hands, life-long, hard-working hands,
hang idle, empty, at his side.

No matter how often he opens and closes his fists,
his mind refuses to grasp fleeting memories.

His brain is swiped clean, as smoothly scoured as
the sand beneath the riling sea behind him.

This is a portrait of a man with
Alzheimer's Disease.

Behold the man!

In reference to the Front Cover photograph, taken by the author
at Nag's Head, Outer Banks, North Carolina.

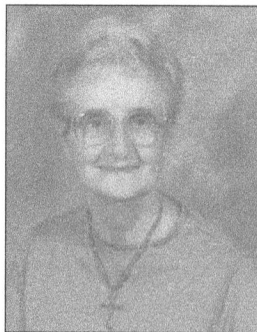

Living, Losing and Learning

Living, Losing and Learning

A Faith Journey from Bitter Grief to Peaceful Acceptance

Cecile R. Bauer

SEABOARD PRESS
JAMES A. ROCK & COMPANY, PUBLISHERS
FLORENCE • SOUTH CAROLINA

Living, Losing and Learning: A Faith Journey from Bitter Grief to Peaceful Acceptance
by Cecile R. Bauer

SEABOARD PRESS

is an imprint of JAMES A. ROCK & CO., PUBLISHERS

Living, Losing and Learning: A Faith Journey from Bitter Grief to Peaceful Acceptance
copyright ©2016 by Cecile R. Bauer

Address comments and inquiries to:

SEABOARD PRESS
James A. Rock & Company, Publishers
1937 West Palmetto Street, #248
Florence, SC 29501

E-mail:
jrock@rockpublishing.com   lrock@rockpublishing.com
Internet URL: www.rockpublishing.com

Paperback ISBN: 978-1-59663-880-8

Printed in the United States of America

First Edition: 2016

For the Warrior Women and Men

Whose Armor is Prayer

When God Claims Their Loved Ones

Too Soon

May Heavently Peace Calm Your Grieving Hearts

The Birthday Party

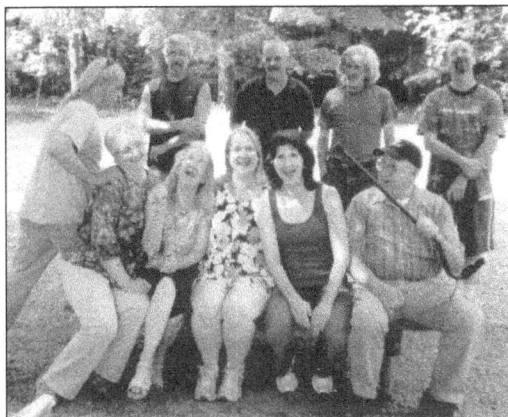

*Davy pushing Cecile (Mom) against Cathy,
Rose, Barb and Daddy Dave.
Back row: Mike, Jason Russ, and Jim*

On my husband Dave's 80th birthday, our oldest son, Davy, and his lady friend Bonnie, arranged a big family party at Chestnut Ridge Park in southern Buffalo. Most of our birth family attended, five of our six sons, and three of our four daughters. We gloried in our big family. Parties and various other joyful occasions were reasons to gather and celebrate. The only missing family members were Tom and Jean, from California. Both sent cards and apologies to Dad for being unable to attend his birthday party.

Jason, from Arizona, and Barb from California joined us at our Pennsylvania home that week. We traveled together to the park. I drove because hubby Dave suffered from mild senility, a brief preview before full-blown Alzheimer's disease. All the western New York family attended. Kids were everywhere, too much food, lots of stories and laughter. At one point, we gathered for family pictures. We lined up our immediate family, Dave Sr., and Dave Jr., Jason, Russ, Mike and Jim, Rose, Cathy, Barb and me for a group photo. Dad and I sat on a picnic table bench with our daughters between us. The guys lined up behind the table, since they were taller than the rest of us. Dad plopped down on the end of the bench. Dave Sr. liked to spread out when he sits, no matter the seat or the occasion. That left the girls and me struggling to find room for our bodies on the rest of the narrow bench. At the opposite end of the bench, my rump was hanging in mid air. Suddenly our oldest son Davy took over. He placed his hands on my shoulder and hip and shoved me toward the girls.

"Move over!" he roared, and pushed us all playfully.

Dad felt the pressure of many bodies shoved against his. He glared around, shaking his cane at Davy. Perfect picture of family fun! Davy pushing hard, the gals laughing (Cathy was laughing like a little girl), and Dad shaking his cane. Our sons stood behind us, all laughing.

Youngest son Jim is staring up at the sky as if to plead, *"Father, save me from this crazy family!"*

Family fun. A perfect day, a wonderful snapshot to cherish forever.

The last day the family unit was complete. Fifty-five days later, our happy family shattered as the first of the deaths began.

> *"And the last shall be first,"* Matthew 19:30
> *Baby Boy, the first one to die.*

CHAPTER 1

Jim (aka, Baby Boy)

James Cecil Bauer, named for his deceased grandfather, was always called Jim by the rest of the world. I called him Baby Boy. As he grew old enough to understand my loving label for him, he hated it! Disrespectful in his young ears. A taunt when he heard it from the rest of the family, especially his five older brothers and four older sisters.

"Mom's calling for you, *Baby Boy!*"

"I'm not a *baby*, Mom!"

But he was my baby boy. My last born, the babe that came along four years after we thought our family was complete. Jim was our bonus baby, the child I thought would be the light of my life, long after his older siblings had grown up and gone on to live lives of their own. Baby Boy. How I loved him, and how he broke my heart again and again.

But in the beginning, he was my heart. The child I cherished and thoroughly enjoyed as he grew from diapers, to pre-school, to kindergarten. Not that we had an easy ride with this precious child. Not at all. Born after 24 hours of labor (maybe he didn't

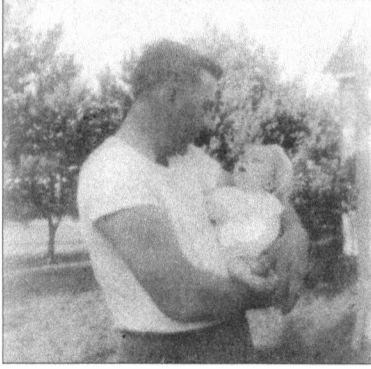

Dad holding Jim as an infant.

want to face the cold cruel world beyond the warmth and comfort of my womb?), he had health problems from his second day. A blood disorder tore him from my clinging arms to a bigger, better hospital fifty miles away in Buffalo. He needed two complete blood transfusions before the jaundice that stained his skin a dark yellow faded into a healthy pink color. Maybe almost losing him so early made him extra special to me. Maybe knowing that this would be my last chance to be a good mother, maybe all that stress and worry helped forge the close bond between us. I don't know. He was always my precious baby boy, and no amount of protest from either Jim or his siblings changed my perception of him as my very special baby boy.

We almost lost him again. He was five months old and a mild cold turned suddenly into a serious pneumonia that put him back in the Buffalo hospital that saved his life previously. I had been working as a school bus driver for the Hamburg, New York school district. After morning runs, I drove immediately to Mercy Hospital and spent the morning with my baby until it was time to drive afternoon take-home bus runs. After that, I would either rush home to fix supper for the rest of the family, or go directly to my second job as a waitress. Daddy Dave stopped every evening after work to check on Jim. One evening, he had great news.

"Doc said we can bring Jimmy home tomorrow evening."

The entire family rejoiced, even Mike, four years old, the former baby, who made no effort to hide his jealousy of the new kid in the family. Mike never liked *anything* new. Not even the new fishing boots that I brought him from the Gaspe' Coast after a second honeymoon with Daddy Dave (he threw them down the cellar steps in protest!) He especially didn't like a new baby "hogging all the attention" in our large and loving family. Mike wasn't in school yet, so our neighbor took care of him the days I worked, or when I spent time with Baby Boy at the hospital. But Mike must have picked up on the worried tension as his siblings and parents stressed over the baby's five-day stay in the hospital. That evening, as everyone rejoiced over the return of Jim, Mike surprised everyone when he gave his little brother a hug.

"Don't be sick no more, OK, baby boy?"

Jim, five months old and not shy at all around anyone, even a resentful older brother, leaned down from Dad's arms and made a grab at Mike's glasses.

"No! Mine!" Mike said.

Everyone laughed in amazement. Mike had fought wearing his glasses with all the stubborn strength of a determined four-year-old Bauer boy. He had thrown the glasses at the wall and broken them so many times that we had a standing appointment at the optometrist to order new frames. One unforgettable day, he had thrown them into the garbage barrel as someone burned the trash. He was not sorry at all. He grinned triumphantly as he rode his tricycle away from the scene of his crime. Enraged, I grabbed him off the toy and tossed the bike into the burn barrel. *Now* he was sorry.

Jim, even at five months, was a problem solver, a peacemaker in our family. One grab at Mike's glasses and, *bingo,* Mike took possession of his long-hated eye-wear.

"No! Mine!"

Baby Boy, the miracle worker.

CHAPTER 2

Mom's Spoiled Baby Boy

When Jim was a toddler, I worked two jobs for the first few years of his babyhood. I drove a school bus for Hamburg schools during the day and worked as a waitress at Holiday Inn four nights a week. One fine spring morning, toddler Jim broke out in spots. Spots as in Chicken Pox. Grandma Bauer, who lived with us for many years, had gone on to her eternal reward when Jim was two. Now, I depended upon a neighbor to take care of Jim between the time the high school kids left for school and I returned home from the bus run. Rather than expose our baby-sitter's family to this pesky disease, I took two weeks off from the bus garage to stay home and take care of my little boy. This turned out to be a wonderful blessing.

It was great to sleep in a bit instead of rushing around, leaving the house before most of the school kids were out of bed. We could actually enjoy breakfast together. I sat at the kitchen table, marveling at the independence of my herd of children. It was like watching a re-make of *Cheaper by the Dozen*. My head spun back and forth as I watched the noisy warfare between the teens arguing about who was hogging the bathroom, and the younger ones making their lunches.

I loved staying home with Jim. He always had this wonderful sense of humor, even as a toddler. Everything he did seemed to make me laugh. *My darling boy.* We had almost lost him twice. To say our youngest son was a cherished child was a serious understatement!

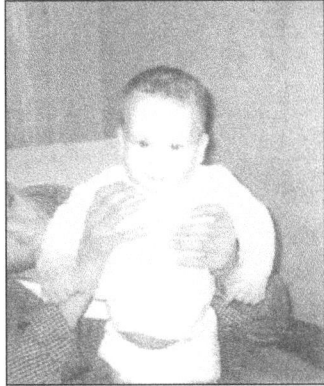

Jim as baby (held by brother Davy).

Toddler Jim and I did a lot of laughing in those two weeks. He was truly a delightful child. Again I learned to cherish every moment spent with my last born son. After two weeks, when Jim was spot free, I called in my resignation to the bus garage.

"I'll come back to work when my boy starts kindergarten," I promised.

"But that's, what, two, three, years from now? You will lose seniority!"

"Oh, well ..." I said. "Family comes first."

My heart sang as I hung up the phone. I grabbed up Jim and did a quick-step around the living room. "Free! Free at last!"

He chortled and clapped his hands. His eyes, which had remained blue until shortly after his first birthday, now gleamed a deep Bauer brown. His strawberry blond hair had darkened as well to a light brown. I didn't care what colors his precious body sprouted, he was still my baby boy. We hugged and danced.

So what did we do with our new-found freedom? Why we went shopping, of course! My car needed two tires (Dave nagged me about it for months it seemed). Funny quirk: I hate spending money for car tires. Always have, always will. But now, to celebrate my newly freed spirit, and because Grant's Department store had a sale on new rubber, Jim and I went tire shopping.

It was a quiet day at Grant's (a store like today's Target). Very few other shoppers lingered in the vast aisles of the store. We stopped first in the auto department, picked out the tires, and then took the sales slip up to the register. Jim was riding shotgun in the shopping cart seat. He held out his arms and cried, "Whee!" as I zig-zagged the cart down the aisle.

"Having fun, Baby?" I said, chuckling.

He grinned, and then suddenly leaned far over the side of the cart. I slowed to a stop before he fell out on his head. I made a grab for him, but he was already out of the cart, running as fast as his little fat legs could carry him. I laughed and raced behind him. *No harm done,* I thought. *No one around to snatch him up and carry him away.* We both came to an abrupt halt in the toy department. I stopped so quickly, the wheels skidded and complained. No worry about hitting Jim. He was already perched on a riding toy. One fat leg on either side of the toy, which moved whenever he pushed his feet along, Jim held on to the handles and beamed.

"Brummm-brummm!" he said, his little face as serious as Mario Andretti rounding the last lap in the Indy 500. "Brummm-brummm!"

"Nice wheels, Jim," I said.

"Brummm-brummm!"

Now remember, this was my last child, my baby boy. What could I do? Deny him a riding toy? Not this Mama! I searched for a price tag. Nothing. A search of the shelves nearby did not display another riding toy for price reference.

"Brummm-brummm!"

"OK, honey. You can have your precious brummm-brummm. But we need to take it up and pay for it."

"Brummm-brummm!"

I tried to pick him up off the toy in order to put it into the shopping cart. Those fat little toddler legs were pretty strong. They wrapped around the toy so tightly, I ended up lifting child and riding toy and plunking them, as a unit, into the shopping cart. At the register, Jim again refused to climb off the toy. He and his precious brummm-brummm rode the register belt together. The cashier grinned the entire time she swiped the bar code into the register.

Who could possibly resist my darling boy and his new toy? He rode it out of the store, through the parking lot, and into the back seat, where I belted toy and boy together for the ride home.

"Daddy's going to be so surprised when he sees my new tires, Jim."

My baby boy could care less about new automobile tires. "Brummm-brummm!"

Did I love Jim too much?

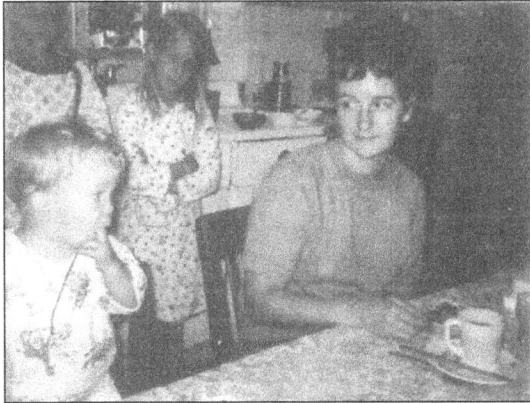

(Front) Baby Jim, the Brumm-brumm lover
and mom, Cecile.
(Rear) Sisters/daughters Cathy and Rose

CHAPTER 3

The Making of an Alcoholic

A mother's guilt knows no time line. Did my smothering love for my last born son make him weak? I could deny him nothing as he grew from a toddler to a teenager. Did my generosity create a sense of entitlement in my baby boy? Did he believe that anything that made him feel good was all right, despite the often serious consequences? These questions haunt me now, as I remember how many times I bailed him out of scrapes, most of them due to his heavy drinking.

From the time he snuck his first drink of beer at a cousin's party, Jim's descent into alcoholism seemed inevitable. He was only thirteen at the time, and his over-indulgence seemed comical at the time. I held his head as he puked. He swore solemnly to never touch beer again. Ever! Yet, despite Jim's vow and this first unhappy experience with drinking, Dad and I noticed beer seemed to disappear from our refrigerator at an alarming rate.

We stopped buying beer. Neither Dave nor I missed our occasional brew. Yet our abstinence did not prevent Jim from finding alcohol elsewhere. Brother Mike had older friends who were only too happy to buy beer for Mike's kid brother. I could list many occasions when Jim got into trouble during his high school years. We always bailed him out. Lingering love for my deceased son prevents me from sharing these unhappy events. Professional counselors have a name for parents like us: enablers.

Jim married at age seventeen, and the drinking spiraled out of control, despite his loving wife, Andrea.

Rear: Jim. Bottom row: Jonathan, Andrea, Bryan

CHAPTER 4

Jim and Andrea

When Jim turned sixteen he earned his driver's license and began to work an after-school job. He commuted to Hamburg on his motorcycle, and worked as a behind the scenes prep-chef at Burger King. Across Camp Road, the Casseri family owned a business, providing jackets for sports' teams and other businesses. Andrea Casseri, a classmate of Jim's, worked at their family business after school. Soon she began to make trips, many trips, daily trips, to Burger King, to buy fries and flirt with Jim. Andrea was and is a beautiful gal. Strawberry blonde hair, big blue eyes, and a movie star figure. Jim had been in love with her since fifth grade. He even earned detention at school one year for trying to reach down her blouse for a freebie touch. She had slapped him then. She wasn't slapping him now.

Andrea was eighteen and Jim seventeen when they got married, a month before their high school graduation. Andrea had lost the baby they expected two months before their wedding, but nothing would deter the young lovers from getting married. Both families, the Casseri's and our Bauer family, tried to discourage such a young marriage, but the kids were determined.

It was a beautiful wedding. The marriage, not so much. Lots of yelling and pouting, and for Jim, drinking. They stuck it out through good times and bad times, rejoicing at the birth of two sons, born three years apart. Inevitably, they began fighting over Jim's accelerating fall into alcoholism. He tried to get sober, and did manage to stay sober for long periods of time. Then another quarrel, a stressful job that kept him on the road for weeks at a time, and Jim would turn to the bottle again. Vodka was his drug of choice. It was almost odorless and invisible when hidden in an empty bottle of Mountain Dew. When I asked him why he kept drinking such a potent brew, he answered.

"Mom, it's a cheap buzz."

After 22 years of marriage, Andrea gave him an ultimatum, "Either quit drinking, or I'm filing for divorce."

Jim chose drinking. Baby Boy drank himself to death.

Why God? Why did you take Jim, the boy of my heart? Did I make the mistake of loving him too much? Are you such a jealous God that you let my baby boy die before he even reached middle age?

It did not occur to me to thank God for sparing all the innocent people my son might have killed while driving drunk. It took me years before I accepted that when God took my son it was a blessing in disguise.

Thank you God for sparing my son from years of jail time, filled with anguished regret for killing innocent people while driving drunk. Jim was so unhappy at his failure to quit drinking. He could not get sober on his own and he was too proud to ask for help.

CHAPTER 5

August 2011, Jim's Death

Jim's drinking accelerated after Andrea threw him out of their home. She filed for divorce, then an annulment in the Church. Despite her newly single state, she did not seem interested in dating again. She did however gladly accept Jim's child support payments, which were so high that he barely had enough cash to pay rent on his tiny house. A childhood friend allowed Jim to live rent-free which proved to be a curse in disguise.

Jim used all his spare cash to buy vodka. His job took him to southern states. Long drives, lonely drives, far away from his sons. Too far to drive home every weekend to maintain any type of relationship with his boys.

Jim drank. Out of loneliness, out of boredom, out of depression. He drinking grew worse and worse. He called me every week from some lonely hotel room, talking for an hour or more, trying to keep up the appearance that he was fine, when even his voice told me that he was drunk. Again. Still. I listened, tried to convince him to accept help, to talk to a priest or attend AA meetings. He promised me he would try to do better. But next week, same thing. Jim staying sober only long enough to do his job, then hitting the hotel room and still another bottle of vodka.

One summer weekend, he called me from a hospital in Virginia. He had been found by police, parked on a bridge, looking over the edge of the railing, ready to leap to his death. *Suicidal.* He was committed to a treatment facility for a week to dry out. He swore me to secrecy.

"Don't tell Andrea or the boys. Don't tell my boss anything."

I promised, because I felt maybe this time he would get the help he needed to quit drinking. After a few days of his boss hounding me for information, Jim relented and phoned his boss to come and get the company truck, parked in a secure location by the hospital security team. Jim had to borrow money to take a bus home.

Safe at home again, Jim was put on medical leave. He had been on methadone, but without insurance, and of course, no money to pay for anti-depressant drugs, he soon used his familiar pain reliever, vodka, to get him through each day. One Saturday, with youngest son Bryan visiting, Jim passed out driving, drifted into a field and hit a tree. Bryan was unhurt. He climbed out of the passenger window and called 911 on his father's cell phone. Jim escaped with a broken wrist and a few scrapes and bruises. When husband Dave and I drove up to visit him, he swore, "Never again. I am done with drinking. I almost killed my son!"

Familiar words from a lifelong alcoholic. If only ... but if only never seems to work for chronic drinkers like Jim. He recovered from his wounds and went back to work. His employer limited him to in-city work. No driving the company truck anymore. Jim felt as if he was being punished, and that's all the excuse he needed to resume drinking again. Finally, in the spring of 2011, Jim called to tell me the bad news.

"Well Mom, they fired me."

My heart felt as if a knife had pierced it. I knew. *I knew!*
That this was the beginning of the end of Jim's life here on earth.
Without a job to keep him occupied during the day, Jim had no
reason to remain sober at all. The first week of August, I received
the phone call I had been dreading. Oldest son Dave, Jr. called.

"They put Jim in the hospital. He looks terrible, Mom. His
skin is yellow and he can barely walk."

Andrea relayed Jim's orders, "Tell Mom not to come see me
until I feel better."

I said, "I don't care what Jim says, we are coming up this
Sunday. What room is he in?"

When we walked into the ICU of the hospital, Jim was in bed
looking wary and scared. I believe he thought I would yell at him.
His legs and abdomen were so swollen, he looked pregnant with
twins. His skin was a deep dusky yellow. His portable urine bottle
on the stand contained a liquid so dark it resembled strong coffee.
I stared at the proof my baby boy's mortality, and had to look away.
Baby boy was dying. The terrible realization turned me to stone.

When I finally met Jim's gaze, I read the knowledge there.
He knew, too. Thankfully, his father, Dave, seemed unaware. I
feared for my husband's heart. He hadn't been well for a long time.
Alzheimer's disease stole more and more of the real Dad each day.
Now 80, he kissed his baby boy (yes, Jim was Dad's favorite son,
too), and cleared his throat.

"Feeling better Son?" he said.

Jim stared at me, then glanced away as he lied to his father.

"Sure, Dad. I'll be out of here before my birthday."

Jim's friends brought him a cupcake to his hospital room to help
celebrate his birthday, August 12th. Dave and I went up a week later
at Jim's request. He had been admitted to Hospice, signed a DNR,
refused kidney dialysis to help drain the excess fluid from his body,
and just plain gave up. I believe our beloved son felt a certain relief
that his struggle with a life crippled by alcoholism would soon be

ended. He accepted his limited time here on earth, and wanted to be cremated when his unhappy life was finally over. During those weeks he was in the hospital, I called him every evening. He asked me to "make arrangements" for him. I called the funeral home in Eden and made preliminary plans for Jim.

That Sunday, we had a family conference. The hospital gave us a large private room to gather and discuss the future. Present besides Dave and me were Jim and Andrea, their teenaged sons, Bryan and Jonathan, two of his sisters, Rose and Cathy, our oldest grandsons Dave and Chris, Jim's brother Mike, and Mike's daughter Stephanie. As the family tried to make small talk and act cheerful, I took Andrea aside. I motioned to the outside hallway.

"We need to talk."

I told her of the plans I had made with Laing's Funeral home. She said, "Oh, Mom!" and started to cry.

"Listen now, Andrea. Dad and I will take care of the expenses. You need to make the final arrangements after Jim is gone."

"What do you mean?"

"You know. The times for the Wake. The funeral Mass. The dinner afterward."

Her pale face looked stricken, as if she was just now waking up to the fact she would soon be a widow. She touched my arm.

"Can I call you for help when the time comes?"

I hugged her. "Of course."

Jim stared at us as we returned to the meeting room.

"So, what do we do now? Find the nearest crematorium?"

I told him the plans "One day's Wake, funeral Mass at ICC (the church our family had always attended in Eden, New York), then cremation."

He shrugged and looked uneasy. "I don't want to put anybody out."

He meant, of course, he didn't want his family to bear the expenses of his funeral.

I touched his arm, the skin so yellow and dry it felt like parchment paper.

"Jim, the family needs this. We need to say our final good-buys. You know, closure?

Finally, reluctantly, he nodded agreement. He was calm, resigned.

The rest of the family not so much.

We took a long time to say good bye to Jim that Sunday afternoon. Dave and I went first. My husband leaned over Jim's pillow and kissed him on the forehead. "Get better soon, son," he said, and swiped at his eyes with a big handkerchief.

Jim stared up at me like the baby boy he had always been to me. He braced himself for whatever harsh words I might use to express my anger or frustration at his failure to "beat that drinking problem." But I could never be mad at my Baby Boy, the beloved son of my heart. So I said something that sounded stupid even as the words left my lips.

"Keep the Faith, Son."

I meant, of course, that I hoped we would meet again in heaven. I squeezed his shoulder and turned away before I blurted out my real thoughts.

I love you son and I will never, ever forget all the joy you brought into my life.

Rose went next. She, my youngest daughter and the most sentimental of any of my children, began to cry as she kissed her little brother. Jim reached up to touch her hair.

"Don't be sad, Rose. I'm not."

Those kind words have sustained me for years now. Knowing Jim felt at peace before he died. *"Don't be sad. I'm not."*

Two weeks after his 43rd birthday, Jim died. August 26, 2011.

It was a Friday morning. I had talked to Jim the night before and he complained that his breakfast eggs sat heavy on his chest all day. It must have been his big old generous loving heart that finally gave out. Andrea called me as I prepared to make peach jam. I sobbed briefly in Dave's arms, then sent him to visit his brother John because my tears always upset Dave and made him angry. It was a sad pattern in our marriage. When bad things happened, Dave did not want to see me upset. If I cried, he got mad and walked away. Maybe he feared that if he broke down in front of me, I would think less of him as a man? So I sent him away and grieved alone.

As I peeled and cut up fruit for jam, Andrea called me a dozen or more times We worked together to make the final arrangements for our beloved Jim. Inside, I was screaming, shaking my fist at the sky, and cursing a heartless God who snatched my baby boy from my loving arms. But in truth, I could not cry at all.

Jim's Wake and funeral passed by in a numb blur. Our family gathered, all Jim's siblings, according to birth order: Dave Jr., Cathy, Russ, Barb (who came from California with her broken wrist in a sling because she wouldn't stop long enough to have it set), Jean, Rose, Jason, Tom, and Mike. Plus the grandchildren and great-grandchildren, too. It was good to have my extended family all together for the first time since the 1970's. They offered such comfort, but I was too numb to appreciate their loving sympathy.

During the Mass, Jim's oldest son, Jonathan read a beautiful eulogy he had composed in his father's memory. During Jon's mid-teen years, he and his Dad had many fierce battles. Jon begged Jim to stop drinking. Jim, deep into his alcoholism, denied he even had a problem and told Jon to stop "putting him down."

"Have some respect for your father!" Jim bellowed more than once.

My son told me several times, "I have two sons. One loves me. The other hates me."

Yet Jon wrote this beautiful tribute to his father and read it in church, with tears streaming down his young face:

"Jim, many of us here remember him as a brother, a son, a cousin, a friend, a companion. I remember him as a father. Dad cared about his family and his friends above himself. Whenever there was a problem with one of his brothers or sisters, he would always lend out a hand to help. When Uncle Russ came back from California, Dad opened his heart and his home and let him live there for several months. I can't count the times Dad helped out his friends and family with their problems, over the phone. I remember one particular time when Dad talked on the phone nearly the entire night to his friend Kevin from California. I don't know what was going on with Kevin personally, but I do know that Dad was determined to help his friend through the hard times.

Christmas and New Year's were the favorite time of the year for Jim. There were years upon years that Dad, Bryan, Mom and I spent putting up trees and piecing together the old train set that went around the tree. We used to have hours of fun seeing how fast we could get the train to go before it fell off the track. Every Christmas we put out deer food with glitter mixed in so that Santa would be able to find where our house was in the dark. There was one year that I fell asleep in the car on the way home from a family Christmas party and Dad carried me in and tucked me in without even letting me wake up.

Trips down to see Grandma and Grandpa Bauer were one of the favorite times that Dad had with his family. We used to drive down to Pennsylvania on the weekends to visit even if there was no special holiday or gathering. It wasn't until later at night that the family settled down and we started a game of Euchre, which was my dad's and my favorite game. There were hours of laughing, teasing, and Grandpa getting mad when someone trumped his ace.

Those weekends were some of the best memories that Dad and I had together.

I want to share with you something personal Dad told me when I was only 8 years old. It didn't mean much to me at the time, but it does now. He told me that when he had his funeral, he wanted me to tell everyone that he felt he didn't do well enough in life. The truth is, he did do well enough, better than he could even imagine. Dad did have his demons, but in all reality, we all do. Nobody is perfect, we're all human. He had a heart bigger than he could imagine.

We love you Dad and we will always miss you. Thank you."

Thank you grandson, Jonathan. I will treasure your loving words forever.

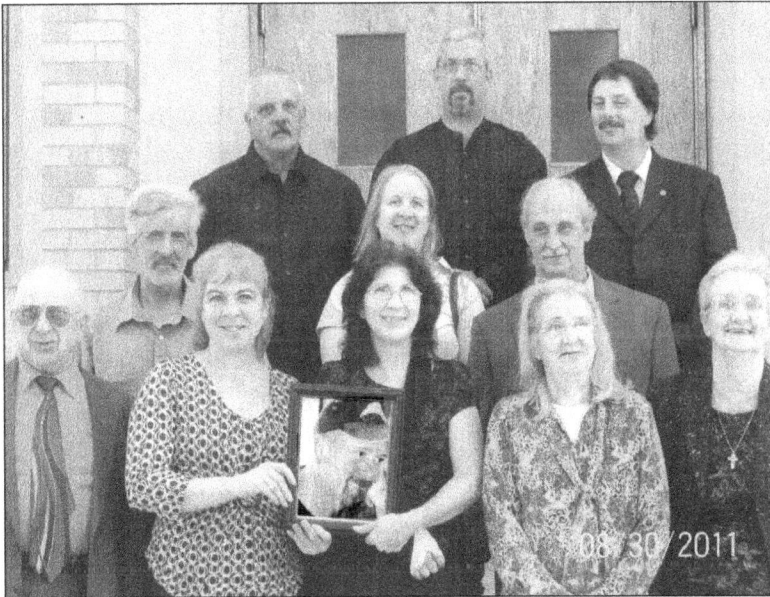

Family in front of church after Jim's funeral.
(Front, L-R) Dave, Jean and Barb (holding photo of Jim), Cathy, Cecile.
(Middle) Russ, Rose, Davy. (Top) Jason, Mike and Tom.

CHAPTER 6

Dave's Tantrum

After a delicious dinner at the church hall in Eden, the family gathered outside, milling around the church steps. Most of the extended family held cameras or cell phones, trying to snap pictures of our assembled family. It had been the 1970's the last time all the Bauer siblings had been together. Several people tried to gather our adult children together for a Kodak moment, but a few were missing.

"Where is Dad? And Rose?"

Grandchildren took off to search the men's room and the social hall for our missing members. Moments later, Rose came outside, holding Dad's arm and urging him down the sidewalk. It was obvious to all that Dad was not a happy camper right then. He was scowling, shaking his cane and dragging his feet, as he grumbled to our youngest daughter, Rose.

"What is going on? How come nobody tells me anything? Dang it!"

Rose murmured something to her father, tugging on his arm and pointing toward the crowd which was waiting, cameras at the ready, to take family pictures. Dave was still grumbling as he walked reluctantly into the middle of our birth family. Our oldest grandson, Dave III, gently lined up the family in front of the steps of the church. Flashes of light, snapping of many cameras, and finally the group photo was accomplished. I have a print of this poignant moment in time, a pausing of our lives during the most difficult day so far, the funeral of our youngest son, Jim.

Our remaining sons, Dave Jr., Russ, Jason, Tom and Mike stand on the steps above us. Daddy Dave stands at the far left, still pointing his cane, mouth open in a mild complaint. But he is half-smiling, basking in the full attention of our large, loving, forgiving family. Our daughters stand in the middle. Barb, her wrist in a soft splint because it is broken and she did not pause to have it set before she hopped a plane from California to her baby brother's funeral, holds a framed picture of Jim. Jean, eyes swollen from tears, stands to the left of Barb and helps her hold the picture. Rose stands a step above her sisters, looking down, embarrassed by her Dad's behavior. Cathy stands beside me, staring off to the side, her face a twisted portrait of grief. As oldest daughter, Cathy felt Jim was her baby too. I stand at the other end of our line of daughters, grinning like a fool, because I could not weep.

After the picture taking comes a time of hugs and good-bye. I receive multiple hugs, grateful for the family love so freely expressed. Dave gives and receives hugs too. Everyone loves Dad's hugs. They are rib compressing hugs, always have been, always will be. I finally break away to get our car. As I pull up beside Dave, he gives me a glare, angry that I am interrupting his hugging time.

"What's the big hurry?" he grumbles.

"Time to go, Dave."

He turns his back to continue talking to our grandchildren and great-grandsons. I turn off the engine and wait. *No use making a scene*, I tell myself, biting back my anger. But my eyes ache with unshed tears and it is a long three-hour drive home. I am exhausted from the stress of the Wake and funeral, the non-restful night's sleep in a strange bed at a local motel. I just want to go home! Jason is watching my face from outside the car. He reads something there that stirs him to action. He takes his father's arm and opens the front passenger door.

"Dad. We have to go now," he says firmly and shoves his father into the seat, cane and all.

Dave does not go easily. He shakes off Jay's hand and shrugs out of his suit coat, flinging it to the ground. Jay keeps shoving until his father is seated beside me. He reaches across to fasten the seat belt. Dad takes one look at his son's determined face and gives in. Reluctantly, he stores his cane beside the console and leans back, crossing his arms in full pout mode. Jason slams the car door, picks up Dad's suit coat, and gives it a shake. A moment later, he opens the back door and climbs inside. He folds the coat and lays it beside him on the seat. Jay meets my eyes in the mirror and smiles slightly.

"Ready to go, Mom?"

I nod and smile my thanks into the mirror.

Many friendly waves accompany our departure. Our family is large and they all long to ease our pain. Dave is too sullen to appreciate this show of family support, but I smile and wave until all are out of sight. I put on the left turn signal and head south. *Going home.*

When we cross the NY/PA border near Warren, I stop for gas. Dave has been dozing most of the way. Now he is awake, still pouting, with arms crossed.

I grab my purse and climb out to pay inside. Jason leaves the car and stands at the pump waiting for the all-clear from inside before pumping the fuel. Dave continues his Buddha imitation. I approach the car and open the driver's door.

"Did you want to drive now, Dave?"

I hold my breath, hoping I haven't misjudged his driving ability. But at that moment I only want to rest without the stress of driving another fifty miles home. Dave reaches for his seat belt. His face is twisted and mean.

"Well, it's about time you let me drive," he says, snarling the words.

"Never mind!" I snap, climbing into the driver's seat and hooking up my belt.

Dave stares at me, his mouth open to curse.

"What kind of a mean trick is this?"

Refusing to even glance his way, I mutter, "I asked you *nicely* if you wanted to drive. But you got all mean and ugly. Forget I even asked. Shut your door! I want to go home."

I feel him staring at me for long moments. If he had refused to come into the car and instead, climbed out, I knew I would throw his cane at him and drive away. Let someone else deal with my stubborn mule. The California siblings had their own car and had left the church yard before us. Jay could text them and someone would come back to rescue their demented father.

Silent rage made my hands tremble. My tiny mustard seed of patience had slipped away, yet again. My face must have been set like flint because Dave finally lifted his leg back into the car, and shut the door. He didn't fasten his seat belt. I never said a word about it. At that moment in time, I truly didn't care if he survived a car accident or not. After a mile or so of the seat belt chiming, he reached over and fastened his belt.

The words I wanted to shout at him sizzled in my mind.

Is this how you act on the day of our baby boy's funeral? The hell with you!

Fortunately, the Holy Spirit whom I credit with all the good words I use, not only in conversation but in writing, kept me mute. If I had let those poisonous words spew out, it would have undone me. I would have wept all the way home.

Forgive me Dave, for my anger that day. And thank you God for tempering my reaction to Dave's deep grief.

Anger is often one of the first steps of grieving. Dave vented his anger on me because I refused to allow him to drive. In his mind, real men drove the car. Wives were delegated to a passenger seat, where, hopefully, they would remain silent throughout any journey. He felt insulted, demeaned, because he no longer had the skills to safely drive the long miles home.

My anger arose from my profound grief over the loss of my baby boy. I needed the strong loving support of my husband. Just when I felt the most vulnerable, he reacted with sullen pouting and shouted words of rage.

Lord, I need loving support, not angry words that make me question my choice of life partners.

Fortunately, we made up our quarrel later that day. Dave never held a grudge. It was not in his nature to brood over past insults or my harsh words. Perhaps that is why his behavior that day was so surprising to me. I realize now that we were both overwhelmed with grief. My grief took the form of silent rage. His grief made him childlike and unpredictable. Not the first time, nor the last that he would have an upsetting tantrum.

Poor Jason, how silently he rode in the back seat. I often caught his worried glance in the mirror as the miles slowly passed. But the fireworks were over, for the time being.

> *God, why am I unable to cry? It feels as if you have torn out*
> *my heart of flesh and replaced it with a stone. Why can't*
> *I shed the healing tears of my profound grief? Am I*
> *afraid of appearing weak before my family? They*
> *all look to me for strength, yet I am weak with*
> *sorrow. I am a punished woman, like Lot's*
> *wife, after I looked back at my formerly*
> *happy family and saw how the death*
> *of our Jim tore us all apart.*
> *I am turned to stone.*

CHAPTER 7

After Losing Jim

The LORD is close to the brokenhearted and
saves those who are crushed in spirit.
Psalms 34:18

After Jim's death, in August 2011, I often found my husband sitting in his recliner, staring out the window. This was not normal for my busy farm boy, especially in the summer when grass needed mowing. When I touched his arm, he would heave a big sigh and turn to me.

"I can't believe he's really gone."

I would nod and turn away.

Baby boy. Gone. Dead? Nooooo!

"Don't be sad. I'm not."

Jim's words of comfort to Rose did not ease my pain now.

"I think of him every day," I told Dave.

I couldn't summon up enough energy to do much of anything those long months after our son died. My writing computer sat idle. Instead of finishing a book in progress, I hit the computer game consol, playing endless games of Spider Solitaire. It took my mind off the real world.

The real world is too painful, too unpredictable, too heart-wrenching. Why are you punishing me this way, O God of all creation?

In my troubled world at that time, I watched helplessly as my companion of over sixty years sank deeper and deeper into his alternate universe. He had three accidents with the car, then forgot how to drive altogether. Of course, he complained bitterly about my driving skills as I took over the driver's seat. We traded in our two vehicles for one car and he complained about that, too. Dave's favorite foods no longer pleased him. The foods he had enjoyed since childhood did not tempt him now. Creamed cucumbers or lettuce salad? Forget it. Fruits? No, only canned pears passed his now finicky lips. Venison, the meat he was raised on and loved better than any other meat? He cut up the steak into little pieces, pushed them around on his plate, and gave them to the dog.

Added to the emotional pressure, our second son, Russ (the Prodigal Son, mentioned in an earlier book), was diagnosed with terminal lung cancer. He lived in the Buffalo area, working for an independent contractor, repairing houses. Russ could do any handyman chore from roofing to drywall installation. But as the cancer grew, his strength and energy waned. His boss took him to a MAC (Mercy Hospital Ambulatory Center) where he was diagnosed and treated under the Hospice umbrella.

I called him every day to keep in touch. The Hospice nurses had both my phone numbers. As the cancer slowly stole Russ's strength, nurses kept me apprised.

"Mrs. Bauer. Russ was found on the floor, cold and unresponsive. The housekeeper got him up again, but he is really too sick to live alone anymore."

I offered to bring him to our home in rural Pennsylvania and use the Hospice Program here. The only problem? Russ had five cats and I am allergic to cat dander. The nurses tried to find homes for Russ's "kids," while I contacted Hospice here in PA.

Meanwhile, oldest son, Dave Jr. and his lady love, Bonnie, did their best to keep Russ comfortable. Bonnie baked treats for Russ. Davy delivered a new television set to Russ. He also paid for cable hookup and the monthly charge to keep TV shows entertaining Russ as he lay in his living room/bedroom. Daddy Dave and I made trips up to visit Russ every few weeks. I took him his favorite childhood candy, circus sponge peanuts.

On Russ's birthday, September 15, 2012, we all assembled at his house in Blasdell, south of Buffalo, for lunch. I had baked a cake and Bonnie made cupcakes. Since Russ loved sweets, he was in heaven that day. The four of us stayed until 3:30 p.m., when it was time to head home.

Davy said, "Want to have supper at Goode's? Bonnie and I plan to stop there"

Dave Sr. and I agreed. We met at the nice family restaurant where we had often dined before. Our dinners came quickly, but Davy had a problem with his food. He had ordered Salisbury steak with double mashed potatoes. His meat was raw and the potatoes cold and hard. We beckoned the waitress and sent the plate back. Much later she returned, but the meat was still raw and the potatoes cold and lumpy. While we waited again, the four of us discussed the unusually bad service.

Our oldest son had never been the most patient person. In fact he had earned the title "Ravy" as a child because of his hair-trigger temper. But as we discussed leaving the restaurant and going somewhere else for a decent meal, Davy surprised us all. He scowled, but kept his angry words to a quiet murmur.

"They must have a new cook," he said. "Young and too dumb to know how to prepare a simple meal."

Bonnie touched his hand. "Want to leave, Dave?"

He shook his head and waited for his dinner. My heart swelled with pride at his calm demeanor. Bonnie had managed a miracle with my oldest boy. She had tamed Ravy's temper.

Finally, Davy received an editable dinner. Later, outside the restaurant, we bid good bye.

Bonnie said, "I guess it will be a long time before we eat here again."

We all agreed, not knowing how prophetic her words would become.

Two weeks later, I stepped out of the shower to answer the phone. It was a little past six on a Saturday morning in late September.

Grandson Dave III told me, "Grandma. Dad died last night."

On September 29, 2012, David Jr. died of a massive heart attack.

Why God? Why did you take Davy now, just when he was so
happy! You know what a tough life Davy had before he met
Bonnie. He was homeless at one point, sleeping in his car,
living in a tent, and so angry at the world. Then he
met Bonnie, and he was finally happy. I don't
understand why You took him now

CHAPTER 8

My Hero Son

He was my firstborn son, David Paul Bauer, Jr., born July 14, 1953. I was barely seventeen while husband Dave Sr. was a young man of 22. We were thrilled and awed by our little boy with the full head of black hair. As I recovered in the new mothers' ward, Dave hurried off to phone my parents, Cecil and Elva Ramier. Most of the new moms in my room had their mothers hanging around their beds, each one cooing over their newborn grandchild. These new grandmothers had been part of the birthing team for their daughters. Holding their hands, encouraging them to push when the time came. Rejoicing with happy tears as a new life entered the world.

I had never even considered notifying my mother as Dave and I climbed into a taxi for the ride to Children's Hospital in Buffalo, NY. Mother and I did not share that type of a close relationship. Her bitter words to us, blurted out in shrill anger after we announced we would need to get married, still stung. She turned away from us. I reciprocated, an unruly teenager clinging to a grudge. If she didn't share our happy news then, why would now be any different?

My parents came to visit the hospital. Pop brought a box of candy and a nice card. Mother brought a handful of flowers cut from their backyard. They both marveled over the perfection of our precious baby boy. Davy served to bridge the chasm of mistrust and hurt feelings that had yawned between the two families. This was Pop's first grandson and he was so delighted, his faded blue eyes glistened with pride. My frozen heart thawed a bit, finally. They even agreed to serve as his Godparents for his Baptism.

Life with a baby sure kept me busy, but it was a happy busyness. I loved nursing my little boy, bathing him, combing his long black hair into a high curl on the top of his head. Even the diaper detail did not bother me. I felt such love for this little boy, so dependent on me! According to the mother wisdom of that time, babies were placed on their tummies to sleep. I kept the bassinet beside the bed. Many times during the night, I would awaken to place my hand on Davy's back to make sure he was still breathing. Because of our low income, we qualified for public housing. We lived in a brand new up-and-down duplex with two bedrooms upstairs.

Davy soon grew into an inquisitive toddler, eager to try new things, a bit of a dare-devil to be sure. A year after his birth, we had a little girl, Cathy, join our family. Now we had two babies in diapers and life really got challenging. An inexperienced wife and mother, I wasted precious energy trying to keep my home spotless. Vacuum three times a week, dishes washed three times a day, laundry put through the wringer three or four times a week, kitchen floor washed every week. Pregnant again, with the son who would be Rusty, my back hurt all the time. It made me cranky, especially since Cathy was a fussy child. Her screams for attention, *right now*, made me bite my lips to keep from screaming back.

One Friday, floor scrubbing day, I struggled to swipe up the kitchen floor before Cathy awoke from her morning nap. On hands and knees, halfway through the chore, my challenging little girl woke up, screaming. Determined to finish the floor before climbing the steps to attend to her needs, I didn't hear Davy crawling up that long stairway. I had taught him months ago how to navigate the steps because he insisted on trying to kill himself by falling down the stairway every chance he managed to slip away from me.

Scrubbing chore finished, I climbed to my feet just as Davy staggered into the kitchen. He carried his baby sister. He held her with his arms around her chest, facing forward. Cathy did not like to cling to anyone while being carried. Her little arms and legs were splayed wide grasping at nothing, face scarlet with outrage, mouth gaping in fear, as her brother hugged her from behind. Davy's face was also red from exertion as he carried the sister who almost matched his weight. How he managed to lift her out of the crib and navigate down that steep stairway without both of them tumbling to the bottom, had to be a miracle.

Dave gasped, "Baby cry," as he handed off his squirming sister into my wet arms.

"What a good boy," I said. "Thank you for taking care of your sister. But next time, let me carry Cathy down those steps, OK?"

He shrugged as if was no big deal to haul his little sister around, whether she liked it or not. He took seriously his role as big brother. All his life, he savored that role. Did not matter that his younger siblings all grew taller than he did. He basked in his role as *boss of all the kids*. He often used his volatile temper to frighten his brothers and sisters into obedience. That was why they called him, "Ravy Davy." The title suited him just fine.

Later, as a married man, and father of two sons, his hot temper cost him his wife. But as a boy, he was so lovable, and so surprisingly funny, that I didn't have the heart to punish him for the hot temper we both shared. Where do you think he learned that savage temper? As a teenaged mom of many toddlers, exhausted and too inexperienced to be a patient loving parent, I often *blew it* too.

After the birth of our fourth child, Barbara, we moved out of the city and into a ranch house in North Collins, a small town thirty miles south of the city. For years, I prayed fervently that God would bless us with a "home in the country." Husband Dave had been raised on a farm, as had both my parents. I felt so safe and contented whenever we managed to visit any of our country relatives. Something about country living speaks to my soul. The fresh air, endless skies, tall trees, big gardens with luscious tomatoes and green onions, apple trees, the whole enchilada.

Dave said it best, "*You might have been born in the city, Honey, but you have a country heart.*"

CHAPTER 9

The Window Caper

The ranch house south of North Collins sat on an acre of land with plenty of room for a big garden. We signed a rent with option to buy contract and moved into our country home just before Christmas 1957. Three bedrooms, a huge living room and roomy kitchen, one bath, all on one floor with a full basement. The boys and girls, two each, shared their separate bedrooms. Life was good, if a little pinched in the finance department. We hadn't budgeted for the extra expenses of Dave's long commute into Buffalo for his job at Firestone Towing company. We pinched pennies, nothing new for our little family. We were always poor in money, but rich in love. Midwinter, we learned another baby would join our family come summer. Budget crunch time.

That was the year I learned to bake our own bread, ten loaves at a time. Chewy, tasty, wonderful satisfying home made bread. We raised our family on that bread.

When spring arrived, it was time to make a garden. Pregnant with Jean, I gazed at that big yard with a sigh. How would I be able to dig up all that wild grass in order to plant a garden? Dave worked long hours, including Saturdays, driving the tow truck. Sundays, we went to church, then he mostly slept the rest of the day.

I sat on the back step one fine spring day, gazing at the grass, trying to work up enough strength to grab the spade shovel and start digging for my garden. Then I noticed a farm tractor, plowing the field behind our property. The man at the wheel seemed young and nice. Did I dare ask a total stranger for a favor? I watched as he plowed row after row, turning over the deep rich soil. On one pass, he tipped his cap at me and smiled. Encouraged, I walked down the length of our property and popped the question.

"Would you mind plowing a few rows for my garden?" I said, rubbing the baby lump under my smock top.

He smiled and nodded. Minutes later, I had the beginning of my first country garden!

I borrowed a tiller from a neighbor and managed to break up the big clods into soil fine enough to plant tomatoes, onions, peppers, lettuce, carrots and peas. My, how good that fresh produce tasted all that summer. Filled our plates and our stomachs too. Tomato sandwiches on homemade bread. Is there anything better?

Of course, gardening is not a one-time thing. Weeds grew and needed to be pulled. Carrots needed thinning. Peas had to be picked every day or they grew too tough to eat. I usually did the garden maintenance while the children had their afternoon naps so they weren't underfoot, "helping," by tromping on the lettuce, sitting on the tomato plants, or gobbling up the fresh peas.

One afternoon, as I pulled weeds, I heard shouting from the house. I looked up to see Davy in the window of the boys' bedroom, yelling at me about something. I waved him away. *Probably telling me Rusty is out of bed, playing with his toys, instead of sleeping,* I thought.

"It's nap time, boys" I shouted, and went back to the gardening.

The yelling continued. Finally, disgusted, I threw down the gardening gloves and marched back to the house. *Somebody needs a spanking*, I thought, fuming.

When I entered the boys' bedroom, Davy had to lean away from the window to see me. His little fingers were caught between the upper and lower window panes. Tears of pain leaked down his face. I rushed to his side to free him from the window's cruel grip.

"Oh, Davy," I said, trying not to cry myself. "I'm so sorry! How long have you been hanging like this?"

He sniffled pitifully. "Only three hours!"

Bet it seemed like three hours, three pain-filled hours, before Mom came to his rescue, ya think? After that day, Davy never tried to open his bedroom window to tattle on his little brother again. This painful experience taught Davy to forge a secret understanding between all my children. They bonded like a wolf pack, them against us. When mischief reared its ugly head, nobody tattled to mom or dad.

Nobody.

Oh the stories they told, as adults, about all the secrets they kept from us!

Thank you, God, for blessing me with a gang of children and happy memories.

CHAPTER 10

Winter Mishaps

In the summer of 1959, after outgrowing our ranch house in North Collins, we moved into a larger house in Eden. Our new home had many wonderful qualities. Big rooms, a two car garage, plus enough space for expansion as our family grew to include four daughters and six sons. We had open land behind us, tall trees for climbing just across the road, and friendly neighbors on either side of our country bungalow.

Best of all, as far as our kids were concerned, were the steep hills holding endless possibilities for a gang of fearless children. In the summer months, the children fanned out over those hills, riding their bikes as fast as their legs could pedal down into the "dip" (their label for the bottom of the steepest hill). Steering around trees and thick blackberry bushes was a requirement, their self-proclaimed "road test" for cyclist. New riders did not always pass this test. Jean, on her first trip down to the dip on her brand new birthday bike, lost control and wiped out.

Davy, always the big brother who felt responsible for his younger siblings, carried Jean home. I met them at the door, alerted by

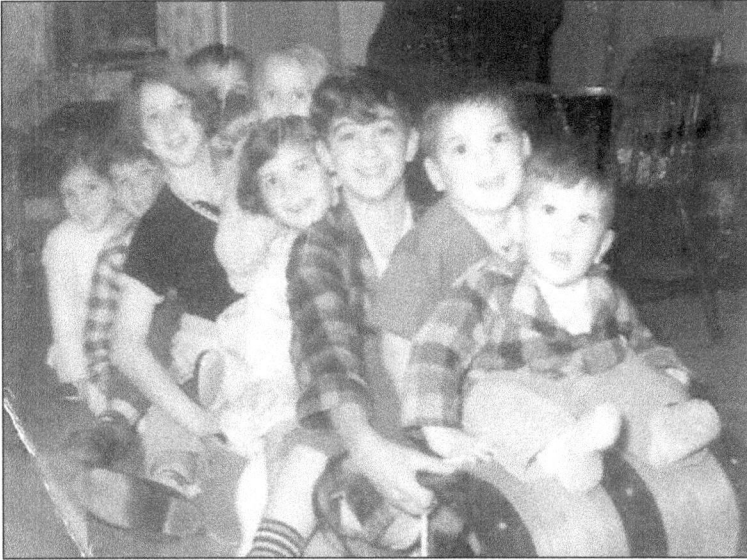

The Bauer Gang on the "Slopes:" Mike, Tom, Davy, Barb, Rose (blonde top of head), Cathy, Russ, Jean, Jason (barely visible top of head).

Jean's howls of pain, and brought her into the bathroom. She sat on the edge of the toilet as I washed and bandaged her scrapes. The sight of all that blood (*my blood!* Jean told me later), made her light-headed. Moments later, she moaned and passed out, falling against me.

"No more hill riding for you, young lady," I scolded as I swiped her forehead with a cold washcloth. But naturally, Jean, as well as the rest of the Bauer children, did learn how to ride safely enough not to wipe out on the steep downhill slope.

In the winter, those hills were transformed into the best playground of all: sled-riding hills. Davy called one "the big hill" because a shallower hill (for sissies) was named "the bunny trail." The big hill witnessed many wipe-outs. Some were just nuisance accidents (hitting a small sapling and being knocked off the sled to cartwheel the rest of the way down without benefit of your sled). Wild rides through the blackberry bushes meant scratches, but nobody seemed to care about that. The best ride, the supreme goal of all the hill riders, was to fly fast enough and far enough to end up in the creek at the very bottom of the dip. They even built snow ramps to increase their breakneck downhill speed. They tried to "catch air', so their sleds flew even faster until someone dropped into the creek. Once this lofty goal was accomplished, all the riders came home, cheering. They helped the half frozen "winner" of the downhill contest as he or she (mostly Davy) waddled, half frozen, into the house. Dripping outer clothing was peeled off and hung on hooks down in the basement near the furnace to dry. Shivering, the downhill daredevil hurried upstairs to change clothing, right down to the skin, because a dunk in the creek meant icy water penetrated everything.

Even some adults, who should have known better, tried out the big hill. My father, then in his early sixties, begged me to accompany him downhill on the kids' new toboggan. I agreed, because, really, it looked like fun to me, too. We shoved off. Part way down the hill, the sled veered to the left and into a small sapling. Both Pop and I rolled off. My father's glasses flew off. I lost my knitted cap. I helped Pop climb to his feet and handed him his snow-covered glasses.

"You OK, Pop?"

He snorted and swiped ice off his mouth.

"That's enough darn foolishness for me."

I agreed, but on another day, husband Dave got the downhill fever, too. It was a mild Sunday afternoon. Fresh powder coated the hills. Davy came with us and surveyed both the big hill and the bunny trail.

"Uh, Mom. Maybe we better do the smallest hill first."

He glanced at his father.

"Snow looks a little hairy for a first-timer."

Daddy scowled. "I've been sled-riding before," he said, bristling. "Why, when I was a farm boy, we used to take out the big bob-sled and ride from the railroad tracks clear down to the lane. Must of been half a mile or more."

"Yes, Dear," I said, "But we were all younger then."

The smallest hill was a short twelve-foot drop from the edge of the field to a former lumber road, no longer in use. The bunny trail was a continuation of the old lumber trail. It gradually curved downhill for 500 feet. The big hill was much steeper, a wild drop of over a thousand yards. We decided to try the shortest hill first and then maybe graduate to the bunny trail.

Davy and I glanced at each other.

"Who wants to be in front?" I said.

Our son grinned.

"That's OK, Mom. Let Dad be first in line this time."

I hid a smile. Even I knew that the front passenger in a toboggan took a direct hit, a face full of snow on the downhill. Daddy threw his booted foot over the sled and sat down in front. I cuddled up to his back. Davy held onto my waist. We pushed off.

As soon as the first icy cold powder hit Dad's face, he reared back, stiffening his legs and pushing Davy and me backwards. Davy laughed loudly, his body shaking against my back, as we slid quickly down that little hill. At the bottom, Dad climbed to his feet, red of face and sputtering snow out of his mouth. Davy dodged away, laughing, as his father took a swing at him.

"So, that's why you wanted me to be first, huh? Should have known it was a trick." Dad grinned ruefully. "Quit laughing at me, darn it."

Davy pointed to the sled trail behind us.

"Wasn't laughing at you, Dad. When you stiffened out your legs, you pushed me off the toboggan. Look, my butt made a trail in the snow."

He laughed again, and pointed.

Sure enough, the imprint of a narrow butt showed clearly behind the stopped sled.

Muttering to himself and still swiping snow off his face, Dad headed home. No more sled riding for my farm boy, ever. But our kids, younger than us and braver, still loved sledding the big hill.

The year Davy turned twelve, our family numbered nine children. Grandma Bauer lived with us then. She was a new widow and her addition to our family proved to be the best thing that ever happened. For one thing, it enabled me to take an outside job to help with the never-ending bills. I worked at Howard Johnson's family restaurant just south of Buffalo, from 5 p.m. to midnight. That meant I was home all day, and Grandma Bauer and I shared the never-ending work of raising a large family. She was a God-send to me and to the children. They raced off the school bus every afternoon, trying to be the first one in the back door where Grandma B met them with freshly baked cookies.

Dave still worked for the towing company and his hours were long and unpredictable. Having an adult in the house to care for the children as I worked at the restaurant gave me peace of mind. Plus the money earned sure helped with the bills!

One busy evening, my boss handed me the phone.

"Call for you, Cecile. Sounds important."

Grandma B sounded upset, very upset. Usually the calmest voice in the house, now her voice shook.

"Davy got hurt," she said, her voice wobbling.

"How hurt?" I asked, struggling to remain calm.

"His knee is all tore up. He hit something, a tree I think, riding that sled down the big hill." She sobbed. "Dave's not home. I don't know what to do."

I bit my lip as I struggled to think clearly. Who could help us? Which neighbor had a car available and wasn't at work, too?

"Mum, send Cathy up the hill to the Nagel's house. Ted will be willing to take Davy to the doctor's, I hope."

I would have telephoned our neighbor but I couldn't think of his number off-hand.

I logged out early at work and raced home. Just as I parked the car in the garage, lights entered our driveway. It was Ted Nagel bringing Davy home. Our wonderful neighbor carried Davy in the house as if he was a toddler. My son looked embarrassed, *being carried like a baby*! But he was relieved when he realized that I did not intend to scold him for his recklessness. His knee was heavily bandaged and already stiff enough to make him limp as he struggled to walk across the kitchen. Mum Bauer blotted her eyes with her apron as she reached up and hugged Ted. Mum Bauer was tall for a woman, nearly six feet, but Ted towered over her.

"Thank you so much," she said. I echoed her earnest statement.

"No problem, Mrs. Bauer. I remember wiping out on that hill when I was a kid, too."

Ted favored Davy with a scowl. "Take it easy on that hill, young man. It can eat you up and spit you out if you're not careful."

Davy hung his head. "Yeah, so I found out."

Ted waved away my offer of gas money for his time and kindness.

"No problem." He tipped his hat. "Evening ladies," he said and walked out the door.

I often wonder if our kind neighbor's warning stuck in young Davy's mind. Probably not. He remained a dare-devil the rest of his life

CHAPTER 11

Davy, Motorcycle Man

After years of riding sleds and bicycles, Davy turned his attention to something bigger and better to satisfy his yearning for, *Speed man. The faster the better.* His first taste of the thrill of riding motorized wheels came on a mini-bike belonging to his friend, Dale Morrison. This was just a little cycle, small enough for a ten year old to ride, but to Davy, it was nirvana, heaven on wheels. Of course he wanted one, too.

I worked two jobs at that time, as school bus driver, and as an evening waitress at Holiday Inn. Davy was old enough for working papers by then, so he worked as pot-boy (dishwasher) in the kitchen. It took him months to save up enough for a cycle, but by fall of that year, Davy owned a full sized motorcycle. He bought it from a friend, a second-hand 250 Kawasaki, fast enough to thrill any rider. Davy, only fifteen at the time, couldn't ride on the road yet but he made up for this by riding all over the fields and wood-paths near our country home. A farmer who lived up the road called to complain about narrow tire tracks through his cornfield. Davy denied doing the deed. I warned him, threatening to hide his cycle keys if he bothered that farmer again. He obeyed. There were plenty of other places to ride his cycle to his heart's content.

About this time, due to the influence of the Beatles, Davy grew his hair longer. No more haircuts from Grandma Ramier (my mother, the family barber for a decade or more). Our oldest son's hair grew long and wild. It had a natural curl that translated to wild frizz the longer it grew. Soon Davy started wearing a knitted cap to bed to keep those curls under control. If he forgot, he woke up with serious bed-head, kinky hair sticking out in all directions like a Brillo pad gone mutant. No amount of pleading or ridicule would make Davy change his mind. He wanted his hair long. Period. About this time he started dodging whenever I approached him. If I dared to reach out and touch those wild but so soft curls, he ducked and ran, afraid I had a hidden pair of scissors ready to attack.

"Gaa Wan! (Go on/get away from me)" he said as he ducked and ran.

I missed touching that soft hair. It reminded me of when he was my infant son, and I could stroke the beautiful dark curls surrounding his baby head. Davy wore his hair long for the rest of his life. Even when his hair thinned and his forehead grew, he kept his hair in a long braid, dangling down his back. He kept riding motorcycles, too.

One day, while riding his cycle, a yellow jacket bee flew up his pant leg and nipped him just below his crotch. Reacting to the sharp sting, Davy pulled onto the shoulder of the country road, dismounted, and dropped his jeans to his ankles. A quick smack ended the bee's life, but the stinger still pumped pain into Davy's thigh. A man of many talents, Davy dipped his hand into the ditch and scooped up wet mud to smear the injury with a mud paste.

"Somebody drove past and honked at me, Mom, but at least my leg stop hurting."

Good old days, indeed. In today's world, Davy might have been arrested for indecent exposure!

When I neared middle age, and the wacky hormones kicked in, I turned to Davy to teach me how to ride a motorcycle. This was a return favor for my teaching him how to drive a school bus. Ford Stamping Plant often had extended lay-offs during the winter months as they re-tooled the factory and geared up for a new model year. Eden schools always needed substitute school bus drivers. Davy loved to drive anything with wheels. After he passed the road test for a bus driver, he often joined me at the bus garage. Davy was very popular with his young passengers. At Christmas time, he returned to the bus garage, his arms filled with gifts and homemade cards. One card made all the drivers laugh. The envelope was addressed simply to "Bus Diver."

"Must be the rough roads, ya think, Mom?" he said, filling the driver's room with his famous raucous laughter.

Later that year, Davy taught me how to ride motorcycles. I wanted to be free to fly down the road on my own cycle. So good to feel the cool air rushing past my face and up under the helmet, eliminating all that bothersome sweat from hot flashes. Not only that, riding a motorcycle saved gas money. As a school bus driver, my four-times-a day-commute, to and from the bus garage, ate up too much gas in my Chevy Nova. Riding my Honda 200, I could gas up once a week for a few dollars. Made sense to me. Plus I loved being a middle aged rebel.

Mike and Jim were in high school then. I used to wave at them as I roared past their school on my way to work. Funny, they always turned away and pretended they didn't know me. I heard later their friends used to tease them about their "Motorcycle Mama." But that never deterred my youngest sons from yearning for their own cycles. As they came of age, they too rode motorcycles.

The summer that Mike enlisted in the Army and did his basic training in Oklahoma, Daddy Dave, Jim and I made our annual trip across the USA to visit family in California. We detoured to visit Mike on the way home. On top of our truck, we hauled Jim's first motorcycle, an old bike made in Japan. Henry, Barb's husband had given it to Jim with a few words of caution.

"It's a good cycle, Jim, but no muffler. So loud, our neighbors complained whenever I rode it. Good luck with your neighborhood."

Jim just grinned.

"No problem, Henry. We live in the country."

Mike, now a different man from the rebellious teen he had been, gazed up at the cycle with real envy in his brown eyes. He ran his fingers through his ultra short buzz cut hair, and sighed.

"Sure hope that cycle is still running when I get my first leave."

After we completed our vacation trip and returned to Eden, Davy came over to the house to inspect and "tune up" Jim's cycle. The bike refused to start at first. But big brother Davy knew a thing or two about stubborn machines and soon had that motorcycle humming. Well, not really humming … more like screaming. Henry was right. With no muffler, the engine roared with a high pitched whine. Hard on the ears. And yes, our neighbors did complain.

But first Davy, as the mechanical genius who made the cycle hum, er, scream, claimed the first ride. He hopped aboard and roared around the house. Around and around he flew, grinning as his long braid streamed out behind him. After the third pass, I held my hands over my ears to block the screaming engine noise. Jim looked alarmed at his brother flew around the house yet another time. He waved his arms to attract Davy's attention.

"My cycle! My turn!"

Finally, Davy coasted to a stop and climbed off the cycle. He laughed as his youngest brother Jim claimed the seat.

"Be careful, little Bro. No brakes!"

Davy turned to me.

"I would have stopped long ago, Mom, but the thing has no brakes at all."

We both stepped back as Jim flew past on his second trip around the house. Jim's eyes were shining. He didn't care if his cycle had brakes or not. He was riding his very own motorcycle, at last.

God, how I miss my motorcycle boys!

CHAPTER 12

Dave and Sue

Davy was twenty and working at the Ford Motor Stamping plant in south Buffalo, when he met Sue. She was young and pretty and fun to be around. Soon they were talking marriage. Sue, just sixteen, was still in high school but she promised to finish her education if both parents allowed the young couple to marry.

They married on November 23, 1973.

Daddy Dave and I rearranged the bedroom assignments in our big house so that the newlyweds had their own apartment upstairs. Next spring, Sue gave birth to their first son, David P. Bauer III. The following year, she had Christopher John. Now a family of four, they moved to a bigger apartment. I missed all of them, especially the babies, our first grandsons.

Married life did not go well for the young couple. Davy, overtired from the shift work at Ford, often lost it in screaming rants, especially if the babies' crying disturbed his sleep. Sue felt tied down by too many responsibilities. She thought her efforts at taking care of those precious little boys went unappreciated by her raving husband. The boys were barely in grade school when Davy and Sue separated and later divorced.

It was a bad time for Davy. Child support payments wiped out his weekly paychecks. He lived on tuna sandwiches and coffee for years, doing without meals in order to buy gas to get to work. Behind on his rent and evicted from his apartment, he lived in a tent all one summer. Daddy Dave and I had moved to California by then and could not offer him even a bedroom to sleep in. One winter he slept in his car parked in the barn of a friend. Later, Mike, home from the Army, and married, offered him shelter in their rented apartment. Long bitter years for our oldest son. He felt such rage for his helpless situation that I feared he might take his own life.

Then he met Bonnie.

CHAPTER 13

Bonnie and Davy

Bonnie. Blonde, soft and comfortable, slight limp from her sore hip, big smile, the kindest heart in the world. That wonderful woman saved Davy. Kind, loving, accepting of not only Davy's fierce rages, but his baggage of staggering debt, Bonnie turned his life around. Together they paid off his debts, saved enough for a down payment on a country home, and became inseparable. Now Davy became a Country Gentleman. He and Bonnie owned ten acres with a barn for Bonnie's horse, Mr. Moe. The house needed work, but Davy thrived on "fixing up my own place." He took early retirement from Ford and spent his days with his precious dogs, his riding toys, Mr. Moe, and best of all, Bonnie.

Bonnie brought out the best in Davy. Her warm, accepting heart grew to include not only Davy and his sons, but also all his younger siblings. They began to host the annual summer party for the extended Bauer family. We all contributed food for the party, but it was Davy who did the grill work and Bonnie who kept the coffee pot going.

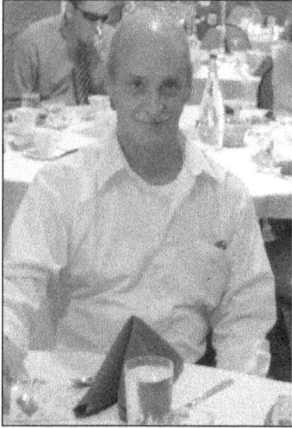

Davy

On Daddy Dave's 80th birthday, Davy and Bonnie arranged to host a big family party at Chestnut Ridge Park in southern Buffalo. Jason, from Arizona, and Barb from California joined us that week. All the western New York family attended. Kids everywhere, too much food, lots of stories and laughter. At one point, we gathered for a picture of our birth family. Davy did his thing, pushing the front row into place while his father shook his cane in protest. The family erupted into laughter over Davy's antics. They shouted in unison, "Gaa Wan!" an echo of Davy's protest whenever I tried to touch his long ponytail.

I treasure that memory and the photo which stands on my dresser beside the bed. Last thing I see before going to bed. First thing I see every morning. Davy, uniting the family.

Davy, as oldest son, made it his mission to help his siblings whenever they needed him.

When Jim fell into tough times after his divorce, it was Davy and Bonnie who went the extra mile. They often visited him, bringing food Bonnie cooked and sharing meals together. The brothers lived just a mile apart, and Bonnie made sure little brother did not go hungry when finances were so tight. They even bought Jim a cell phone with enough minutes on it so he could keep in touch with the rest of the family. When Jim lost his job and deteriorated into fatal alcoholism, it was Davy and Bonnie

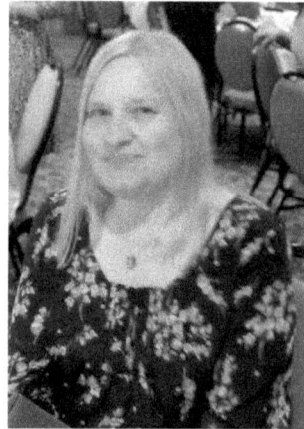

Bonnie

who notified me of Jim's final hospital stay. But even before that unhappy situation, I began to call Davy my hero.

Davy helped all the people he called friends, not just his immediate family. Whenever raucous parties turned people into roaring, staggering inebriates, Davy assigned himself the title of DKK (Designated Key Keeper). Many a wild party animal turned into a sheepish guy sleeping on the couch or walking home because Davy refused to hand over their car keys until they sobered up. Nobody challenged Davy for their keys. He may have been short in statue, but he was one tough dude.

Under Bonnie's gentling, Davy's warm heart emerged. I had wonderful emails from him, describing his new life in the country. One winter a fawn, rejected by his mother, took up residence in his barn, sleeping on a pile of Mr. Moe's hay. Davy put out extra feed for the young deer, careful not to spook it with human touch. One morning he noticed the fawn could no longer stand up. Careful observation showed an infected hoof.

"Mom, the poor thing must have been in so much pain, but it let me wash his foot and pour on some antiseptic."

The hoof did not heal. Finally, seeking help for the wild creature, Davy called the Game Warden. A man came out, took one look at the beast, and drew his weapon. Before Davy could protest, the officer shot the fawn to "put it out of its misery."

Heartbroken, Davy returned to the house and slammed the door.

"Mom, if I had known how cruel that guy was, I never would have called him. Imagine, shooting that young deer and just leaving it in the ditch for the garbage man to pick up. Inhumane! After he left, I went out and buried the fawn myself. It was the least I could do for a creature who trusted me enough to sleep in my barn."

My tender-hearted son. How I miss his great heart and his raucous laughter. Rest in peace, my hero son.

"Live your life so that the fear of death can never enter your heart. When it comes your time to die, be not like those whose hearts are filled with the fear of death, so that when their time comes they weep and pray for a little more time to live their lives over again in a different way. Sing your death song and die like a hero going home."

                                    —*Tecumseh, Shawnee Chief*

CHAPTER 14

Early Morning Telephone Call

Early Saturday morning, September 29th, 2012, the bathroom phone rang. I had just stepped out of the shower. My heart gave a little leap of fear. Russ had been in Hospice care in the Buffalo area for months. Only Hospice would call me so early, I thought. Wrapping the towel around me, I picked up the phone and sat down, dreading to hear the nurse's voice telling me that Russ had died in the night.

"Grandma? It's Dave III."

"Hi Dave! Are you and your family coming down to visit?"

I smiled, anticipating good news instead of bad.

"Uh, Grandma, Dad died last night."

My heart flipped. "What? What are you saying?"

"Dad died last night. He was in an ambulance going from Lakeshore Hospital to Mercy in Buffalo. Massive heart attack, I think they said."

I had trouble understanding my oldest grandson's tearful voice

"Your father? My son Davy? Died?"

My lips went numb. I shivered in the overheated bathroom. Dave III told me later that I hung up on him. I don't remember. Can't remember how long I sat there either. Towel wrapped around my shivering body, I could not seem to make sense of anything. Don't remember throwing on some clothing. Can't remember what I said to my husband Dave to convey this terrible news.

Davy? Dead? Can't be. Not another son taken away too soon. God! Why?

My heartbroken anguish turned me to stone. The following days passed in a numb blur. Barb and Henry, Jean and her son, Nathan, and son Jason, all flew in from the West Coast for the funeral. Dave III and Tina hosted a family get-together that Sunday, but Daddy Dave and I did not drive up to New York that day. I simply did not trust myself to drive over a hundred miles in my state of stony numbness. Husband Dave could not be trusted to drive anymore, either.

We drove up to Eden later that week for Davy's Wake and funeral. Same funeral home, same ultra nice mortician we had trusted to take care of our youngest son's remains, now took care of our oldest son. When we walked into the funeral parlor, Bonnie stood beside Gabe Johnson, the funeral director. I hugged Gabe first.

"We have to stop meeting like this," I told him, choking down a sob.

I wasn't trying to be funny. I meant that our family had too many deaths already, and we all knew Russ would be next.

Bonnie hugged me tight.

"I'm so sorry," I told her. "You don't deserve this. Especially now, when Davy was so happy with you."

"Me, too," she said, wiping her red eyes.

We sat down and she told me what happened the night Davy died.

"We had supper. He only drank one cup of coffee because he had heartburn. He took his shower, went out and walked the dogs, and put down hay for Mr. Moe. He kept walking around outside like he had forgotten to do something. When he finally sat down beside me on the porch steps, he heaved a big sigh."

Rubbing his chest, Davy said, "I think you better call the ambulance. This feels like more than heartburn."

The local ambulance took Davy to Lakeshore hospital, a fifty-mile trip. It would have been more prudent to drive straight into Buffalo, another ten miles by a different route. At Lakeshore, they gave him a clot-busting drug by injection. But Davy's pain only got worse. The attending doctor ordered another ambulance to transport Davy to south Buffalo's ECMC (Erie County Medical Center). On the way, Davy crashed in the ambulance. It headed to the nearest hospital, Mercy, but it was too late. Our oldest son died en route.

When I think of it now, Davy, the blustery, never let them know you might be scared, of anything, oldest son, I have to weep. I always knew inside all that bold swearing and loud yelling beat a heart that often felt frightened by the *real world*.

How scared he must have felt as his life slipped away. Isolated in the speeding ambulance, without any family or friends to hold his hand as his big loving heart gave up. I pray Davy saw the hand of Jesus as Our Lord smiled and lifted Davy into the eternal light.

As I stood beside his coffin, later that evening, I reached out to touch that wonderfully soft hair. I wished vainly that I had a pair if scissors to save a curl or two for his memory book. At the thought, I almost expected him to recoil and duck away from my tender touch.

"Gaa Wan!"

I have no memory of where we slept overnight. Nor of the funeral Mass. I do remember the mourner's brunch because I got lost driving from the Eden church to the VFW in Gowanda. A funny story, but I could not see the humor of it then.

Gowanda is a very small town community. I am as familiar with those streets as I am of the town where we raised our family,

Eden. But somehow, driving south on route 62, I failed to see the familiar sign for the VFW and drove instead onto the main drag and pulled in opposite the Tim Horton restaurant. Our good friends, Ed and Kay, from our church in PA were following us. They pulled up beside our car.

Ed smiled and said, "Are you lost? Because I know where the VFW is. Saw it on the way down the hill back there."

Frustrated, confused, and half mad at myself for not being in control of the situation, I could only nod, and agree to follow my visiting friends (who did not know the area like I thought I did!), to the hall where Dave III and Tina had arranged to host the mourners' brunch. My family teased me gently.

"Mom, how could you get lost in Gowanda?"

We all laugh about it now, but I could not laugh then.

My son, the hero. Dead at age fifty-nine.

Just when he was finally so happy! It's not fair, God.

It is only recently, as I surrender to God's will for my life, that I learned God's plan is always better than mine. Our Lord took Davy at the very best time of his life, when he was completely happy with Bonnie. If Davy had died a few years before, when his wretched life had reduced him to a bitter homeless man, dependent on friends to feed and house him, our oldest son might have committed suicide. But our merciful Father waited until Davy was finally happy, before lifting him into eternal bliss.

I still miss him every day. His grave marker in our family plot in St. Mary's cemetery is highlighted with a motorcycle.

Ride on, my hero son, Davy.

CHAPTER 15

Tina's Tribute

Dave III's wife, Tina, really loved her father-in-law, our son Davy. Originally, she planned to eulogize him at his funeral, but heartbroken, she put this beautiful tribute away for three years before posting it on Facebook.

"David Bauer, Jr.: As we approach the third anniversary of your passing, I'd like to share what I wrote. I have had this tribute since that fateful day, but emotionally was not able to read it at the funeral. Much love to you always.

The oldest son ... one of ten ... I have heard those words many times over the past few days. I started to think about them and wonder do people know what that means? The first thought that comes to mind for me is an enormous sense of humor. Enormous because when he laughed, it was a loud, booming laugh. It was never a soft chuckle or smothered giggle. It came from the belly and was let loose.

What about his gift for telling a story? Do those words above reflect how the man could tell a story? It wasn't just

*a quietly-told event. Oh no, it was sound effects and body
motions and a loud voice with all the emotion of the event
in it. The sound effects were especially entertaining when
they included any type of engine. I still hear it in my head
as I write this. The revving of the engine, how it sounded.
Then there was his body motion. A good story was never
told sitting down, but standing and moving.*

*On the flip side, with that enormous sense of humor,
came the enormous temper. One story comes to mind. It
was the first time I went to his home to be introduced to
him. We walked into his place in Derby and the first sight
that greeted me was a pile of white plastic, little plastic
pieces in a neat pile. As he came out of the bathroom, he
looked at me with his sheepish smile and red face to explain: the (lawn) chairs got in his way. My thought was,
note to self, stay out of his way. I also think I fell in love
with him a little that day.*

*Of course there was the swearing when working on any
type of motorized "toy" from cars to lawnmowers to snow-
mobiles. I would sit and listen and stifle my laughter, but
boy was his face full of expressions.*

*The most important side to him, the one that most didn't
know, was his deep and abiding love of family and friends.
He made it seem like no big deal (his helping others) and
brushed it off, but when he loved, it was without conditions.*

*I remember when his son, Dave III, and I got married.
I climbed out of the limo at the church and saw him standing there in his tuxedo looking so handsome. I immediately
went up to tell him how great he looked, when I happened
to glance down to see he had on these old ratty, velcro
sneakers. I wanted to cry. So I calmly look at him and
ask if there was a problem with his (rented dressy) shoes.
He looks me dead in the eye and with that little grin, says
that he doesn't want them all dirty and scuffed up before
the wedding. I look around the blacktop church parking*

lot and the beautiful sunny day and it hit me. He wants to look good for his son. He was so proud to be there in his tuxedo and he wanted everything to be perfect. It was then that I fell completely in love with my father-in-law.

While going through pictures at his house after his funeral, I found his copy of our wedding invitation and tucked inside was the dried corsage he was given as father of the groom. We also came across every letter, card and gift he was given by those closest to him. Pictures were tucked everywhere, mementos of a life filled with love and laughter.

I am sure everyone could add pages and pages to what I have written. I could write many more stories and wonderful memories, too. I am so happy Dad Bauer found his piece of heaven here on earth before being called home. He had his house and barn in the country, and most importantly, found a deep and lasting love with Bonnie. He was so happy and peaceful on his little farm. This thought brings me happiness that he found it, but equally sadness that he isn't here to enjoy it longer. So, yes, he may have been the oldest of ten children, or one of the ten, but to those of us that have had the privilege to be called his family and friends, he was one in a million and irreplaceable.

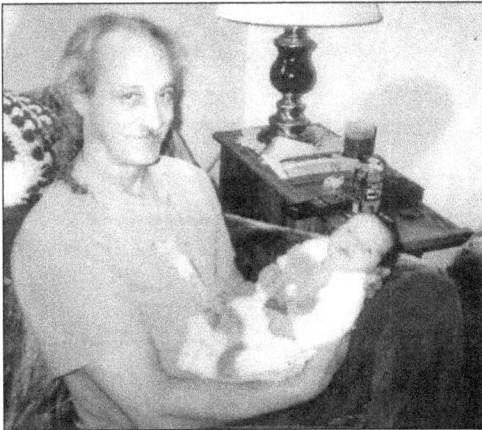

Davy and grandson, Devin.

Well-written Tina. Thank you for loving our Davy with your equally big heart.

CHAPTER 16

Russ's Story

Russ was the son who disappeared from the family for thirty years. After fathering a child in the 1970's, he ran off to California to escape paying child support for his son, Tony. The child's mother refused to marry Russ, and also refused to give the boy his last name on his birth certificate.

Russ said later, "I thought, 'if she won't let him have my name, then she sure isn't getting any money from me either.'"

Selfish? Oh yes, a lifetime of thinking only of his needs and wants went into this decision to squirm out of accepting responsibility for his son. Typical of Russell, third born child, always quiet, always stubbornly refusing to do anything he didn't want to do. A challenging child from the beginning. As a young toddler, he didn't make much of a fuss about anything. Russ's quiet rebellions went unnoticed in our family that included three children under the age of three. Davy and Cathy worked like a team, picking up the toys Rusty played with but refused to put away. He would sit on the rug, thumb in his mouth, dreaming of a world where no one would ever ask him to do anything he didn't want to do, ever!

Rusty's birth was long and difficult. His head was positioned face first in the birth canal, instead of tucked under, crown first, as most babies are delivered. His brain might have been damaged by a lack of oxygen as my long painful labor produced no results. Finally, the doctor gave me a sedative and used forceps to deliver our third child. Maybe the delivery was botched in some way. Whatever happened, Rusty was slow to develop.

Slow to sit up, slow to roll over, slow to walk. Even slower to talk. He didn't *need* to talk. All he had to do was point at something and grunt and Davy or Cathy would fetch it for him. After younger sister Barb was born, a year after Rusty, I finally noticed how much this little tyrant was getting away with on a daily basis. Now four children vied for my attention. One of them was getting a free ride! Totally unacceptable to me, a novice mother at age twenty.

What did I know about training and gently encouraging a mule-headed little boy whose passive-aggression stymied my every effort? Oh, the epic battles we fought! Rusty's stubbornness matched mine. He *would* pick up his toys. He *should* be talking by now. He *needed* to be out of diapers.

Actually, potty training Rusty was not that difficult. He watched, with interest, how older brother Davy raced into the bathroom and did his business with a certain jauntiness. Davy was Rusty's hero, always. Soon Rusty spent regular intervals on the potty chair, sitting passively until he succeeded. He didn't mind being there. Got him out of the toy pick-up detail, right?

One Friday, bathroom cleaning day for me, Rusty strolled into the room and pushed down his training pants. I continued my work, scrubbing out the tub. I heard Rusty coughing. Glancing his way, I noticed tears streaming down his cheeks.

"What? Why are you coughing like that?"

He didn't answer, just gagged and coughed. The sharp smell of bleach stung my nose. I had poured a cup full into the potty. It foamed up, activated by Rusty's urine. Scrambling to my feet, I lifted Rusty off the chair before the fumes overwhelmed both of us.

I laughed as I wiped his face with a cool washcloth. He didn't think it was so funny.

"Oh, Rusty. I'm sorry. I forgot about the bleach I put into your potty chair."

Even my apology did not soothe his wounded pride. He pouted for the rest of the day. So it went with our third-born child.

People outside my immediate family thought Rusty was a wonderful boy.

"So quiet and good," my mother raved.

Pop had another opinion. "The kiddo always has a troubled look on his face."

I called it pouting, but my father looked deeper into Rusty's big brown eyes. I did not understand then that Rusty needed extra attention from me. He was slow at everything. I had no patience for a child who dragged his feet when I needed to get things done, *now*! It took oceans of my limited energy to get Rusty to do anything he didn't want to do. I worried that he would never succeed in school, never apply himself to the simple act of learning to read and write and do numbers.

To my surprise, Rusty loved school. He went off every morning, carrying the lunch he made himself, singing as he climbed on the school bus. How the teaching nuns accomplished what I never had been able to do completely mystified me. What secret did they use to motivate him? Later, older and wiser, I realized that the nuns shared what they are famous for: lavishing love on every child in their care. I never learned that lesson in time to help Rusty. He grew up without either of us ever really connecting on any emotional level. I was Mom, too strict, too demanding. He was Rusty, too quiet, too stubborn, isolated from the rest of our family. In a gang of rowdy kids outgoing and eager to please, Rusty grew up sitting alone and watching, without joining in on the really fun stuff.

While his siblings shouted and slammed their sleds down the big hill, Rusty came home early. He hated being cold. When Grandpa came to visit on a rainy day and went outside with the kids to splash in the puddles, Rusty stayed inside. He hated getting wet, too. Yet one memorable day, a neighbor called to warn me.

"Your little boy is outside, walking in his bare feet on the roof of your porch!"

Yep, walking in his bare feet across twelve inches of fresh snow. He had climbed out the bedroom window upstairs and ventured to the edge of the porch roof. What happened to the guy who hated the cold and snow? He climbed back into the bedroom when I beckoned. A small smile of triumph curved his lips as I turned him over my knee.

Later, when I grew older and wiser, I realized, too late, that my mule-headed third born child had discovered a sure way to get Mom's attention: *act up*. What better way to insure a busy mother's full attention than by doing something so outrageous it put his life in danger? I missed the crucial sign that Rusty needed more than my casual glance as I rushed from chore to chore, child to child. He used that newly discovered knowledge as only a rebellious child can do: by getting into as many scrapes as possible.

At the time, frightened by Rusty's reckless actions, I made sure Daddy Dave fixed that bedroom window so it wouldn't open again until our puzzling son learned not to endanger himself by crawling outside on a bitterly cold winter day.

Life continued on, life with a reckless child, who hid his intelligence under the cloak of "I don't care." He did take a stand about one thing. At age ten, he demanded we now call him Russ instead of the childish Rusty nickname the entire family called him. Maybe it was because he hated the label his sisters and given him? *Crusty Rusty*. His sisters, being female and mini-moms in the making, hooted and laughed whenever their brother took a much needed bath (he hated water, even nice warm bath water). Because he used every excuse possible to avoid bathing, when I finally cornered him and insisted he, "Take a bath! Now!" Russ needed a Brillo pad to lift the ground-in dirt on his knees and elbows.

Crusty Rusty. No wonder he demanded we now call him Russ!

When he was twelve, he took a diving leap out of a pine tree and broke both his arms. I think he believed his injuries would save him from dish drying duties. During that time, with a houseful of children to help out, we had posted a schedule with teams of washers and driers to help with meal clean up.

As our family doctor put casts on both arms, Russ smiled with relief. But no, despite his protests, he didn't miss his turn drying dishes. It took months, years, before Russ finally, grudgingly, accepted some responsibility for his actions. But it remained a battle right into his late teens.

CHAPTER 17

Banishing the Prodigal

Cleaning his pigsty (room) one day, I found drugs hidden in
his things. He denied they were his. When confronted with proof
(a homemade pipe in his dresser, baggies under his mattress) he
tried weeping to escape my anger. Didn't work. Finally he admitted
the drugs were his and vowed to quit the habit. Promises were
always a challenge for Russ. He may have meant well at the time,
but "Mom, they made me feel so good."

Feeling good seemed to be what my second son valued most
of all.

At age twenty, high on weed, he risked his brother Tom's
life in a game of chicken on the road out front of our house.
Screeching brakes alerted me to their dangerous game of
life or death. That ended it. I threw Russ out of the house.
He was twenty, old enough to survive on his own. No more
drugs in our house. No more risking a sibling's life just for
the thrill of it.

Years later, when Russ returned to the family fold, he gave both
Daddy Dave and me little glass statues as peace offerings. Dad's

was an eagle with outspread wings. Mine was an angel with its arms reaching out. Russ told me what the angel represented.

"It means all is forgiven, Mom."

Excuse me? Russ is forgiving me? What about all the trouble he gave the entire family down through the years? I thought about telling him where to shove his statue, but age and wisdom kept me mute. Russ was back in the family. Maybe he had learned something, in the cold cruel real world, during his long sojourn on the West Coast.

It took months before Russ and I could communicate without accusations tossed back and forth. He camped with his brothers in western New York until he finally moved into his own place. The brothers wanted to help Russ, but his general laziness, plus his five cats, made him an unpopular guest for any longer than a few months. These were the youngest brothers, Jim and Mike, who had been too little to remember their older brother before he left the family fold. Now years later, when Russ moved out, both siblings breathed a big sigh of relief.

Russ worked as a helper to an independent contractor, fixing up houses. He was skilled at all jobs from roofing to flooring to wiring and plumbing. Finally feeling independent, he began to telephone me and brag a little about his success. It took a few months, but we finally began to connect as two adults, instead of mom and rebellious son. He was in his fifties now, and seemed contented, at last, in his little rental house with his five "kids," the cats he brought with him from California. I enjoyed our conversations, appreciating the effort he put into call me on a regular basis. One evening, during a phone conversation, he surprised me with good news.

"Guess what, Mom? I started going to church again."

Wow, major step up into mature adulthood. He admitted that when we gathered here at home and said Grace before meals, he barely remembered the words he had recited along with his siblings for fifteen years.

Thanks God, I thought. *Finally, there might be hope for Russ yet.*

During the winter of 2011, the building trade slowed down and Russ had money problems. He hated to ask, but could I help him with his electric bill before they shut off his heat? Of course I sent him a check for that month and for all the winter months after. Couldn't have a child of mine freezing, could I?

That following summer, Jim died. Russ attended the Wake and funeral in a new shirt that looked too big for his narrow shoulders. When I asked him about the obvious weight loss, Russ told me he was working too long and too hard to stop to eat. I scolded him, of course. That's a mother's job after all.

"You can't starve yourself, Russ, and keep working so hard. It will catch up with you. Your body needs food to thrive."

"Yeah. Yeah!" An echo of his teen years, come back to haunt me.

The winter of 2012, Russ called me late one evening. He sounded scared.

"Mom, my boss took me to the MAC (Mercy Hospital Ambulatory Center)."

I heard him swallow hard.

"What? Why?" I said.

Russ had been complaining of a bad cold that made his chest hurt whenever he coughed.

"They took X-rays, Mom." Another long pause.

"And? What? Just tell me, Russ."

"The doctor said I need to go to the hospital! But I don't have any insurance. How will I pay for a hospital visit?"

His voice rose in a shrill fear that told me he was afraid of more than the thought of a future hospital bill. I drew a deep breath and tried to remain calm.

"Russ, every hospital treats people whether they can pay for it or not. Federal law."

"But ..."

"No buts about it, Russ. Go to the hospital. Will your boss drive you over?"

"Doctor says I need an ambulance."

My heart sank. I think I knew then that Russ's chest pain was more than a simple lung infection. Doctors don't request an ambulance to transport a simple case of pneumonia.

Much later that night, at midnight, Russ called me from the hospital.

"They're keeping me here, Mom."

He wouldn't tell my why. His voice sounded scared and defeated as he gave me his room number so I could contact him the next day. After a sleepless night, a long night of prayerful pleadings to God for mercy and healing for Russ, I talked to my son again.

"Yes, Mom. They told me it is lung cancer. Stage 3.5, whatever that means."

I knew what it meant but kept the knowledge to myself. Russ was already scared. No use making him worse. His next question made my heart sink like a heavy stone.

"Mom, what is Hospice?"

"Hospice is the best thing that can happen to you right now, Russ. It means doctors and nurses will come to visit you at home, instead of you driving to their offices. It means your medicines will be paid in full, and delivered to your house, too. No charge! It is a wonderful program. Grandma Ramier had it when she developed lung cancer."

He took a deep breath as he mulled over the cruel facts.

"Grandma died, right?"

"Everybody dies, Russ. Some sooner than others."

"Like Jim, right?"

My turn to take a deep breath.

"Yes, like your brother, Jim."

"The nurse is here," he said abruptly, and hung up.

Russ signed the papers for Hospice that day. He seemed resigned, no longer so frightened, about his limited future. But Russ was always a tough read. I never knew for sure just what he thought or what scared him spit-less. Our daily conversations continued. As he sank deeper into a drug-induced calmness, he did not always make sense on the phone. He needed stronger and stronger pain medicine to take the edge off the deep pain in his chest. Friends moved his bed down from the second floor of his rental house to the living room. He slept sitting up and needed oxygen to ease his raspy breathing. Nurses and housekeeping people came every week to take care of him. I felt helpless, unable to really help him, because we lived so far away.

Daddy Dave and I drove up to visit Russ every few weeks. I brought him books to read and his favorite childhood candy. It seemed so little to do to help a dying man. We could never stay more than a few hours because Russ's five cats really did a number on my lungs. The visits always ended the same. As I hugged Russ goodbye, I tried not to look at him too intently. He might guess that I was memorizing his face in case I never saw him alive again. One week, after coming home, I telephoned the same mortician who had handled Jim's funeral. We made tentative plans for Russ's demise.

Two sons. Two sons dying too soon.

I stopped praying for healing for Russ and began to pray for a swift merciful death. Even Daddy Dave (suffering from early Alzheimer's disease and pretty self-centered these days) noticed how weak and frail our son had become, and how much pain he suffered.

"I feel bad for Russ," Dave said as I drove the long road home.

I reached across and patted my husband's knee. Neither of us needed to say what we both knew: Russ's days on earth were limited.

Hospice nurses called me frequently. They were pushing for more family involvement for Russ. His brothers, nieces and neph-

ews, and his son, Tony, all visited him. But no one could take time
out of their working lives to move in and take on the big job of
caring for a dying man. I offered to move Russ home with us, but
told the nurse frankly about my cat allergy.

"Russ is welcome to live here and I will gladly take care of
him through Hospice, but I cannot deal with five cats. Not even
one cat."

His primary nurse heaved a long sigh, and promised she would
try to find good homes for Russ's feline kids. True to her word,
the nurse called me and we both rejoiced that we could now take
on Russ's care. Two weeks after son Davy died, we moved Russ
home with us.

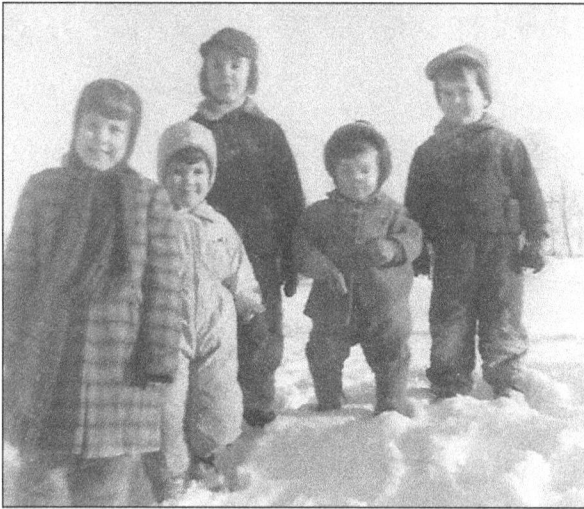

(L to R) Cathy, Barb, Davy, Jean and Rusty

CHAPTER 18

Home at Last

Mid-October, 2012, Daddy Dave and I drove up to Russ's house to bring him home with us. It took all day to load up the big trailer. Several Hospice nurses and one of their chaplains helped us. Russ sat in his battered recliner, oxygen tube in his nose, and watched as we buzzed around him. The biggest problem for all of us was what to take and what to leave behind. Our sick son had a large collection of odds and ends. Numb from pain killing medicine, he seemed unable to decide what he wanted to keep and what could be discarded as useless junk. In Russ's eyes, everything he owned was precious, even the rough horse blankets, so loaded with cat hair to be unusable. He wanted everything moved south. Finally, Dave and I did the weeding out of what was usable stuff and what to leave behind as junk.

Russ insisted we take his oak table with a nice big leaf, plus his cedar chest (filled with hair-covered horse blankets). He wanted all his working tools, too, and maybe the television set. Finally, struggling to decide what to take out of his refrigerator and freezer and put in our large picnic cooler, and what should be abandoned to the house owner, I put my foot down.

"Russ! The trailer can only hold so much. We can't take everything you own. Make your decisions. Now."

I glanced over at my scowling husband.

"Dad is already tired out. We need to load up and start home before dark."

We took his tools, a few clothes (most were not worth saving), the table, the cedar chest, and his bed. We filled in the scant spaces in the trailer and the back of our SUV with whatever Russ decided was vital to his waning lifestyle. This included two tanks of oxygen, and his walker.

Dave, truly worn out, took one look at the lop-sided trailer (loaded by the chaplain), and sighed. Without another word, he unloaded everything and started over. Obviously, the chaplain had never moved furniture. Miffed, the man left. Dave and I reloaded the trailer into a balanced load that wouldn't tip over halfway home. It was after 4 p.m. before we finally pulled out of Russ's driveway. A bit later, we stopped at a fruit market and bought sub sandwiches for supper. Dave had driven from Blasdell to Hamburg. After our supper stop, I drove the rest of the way home. About an hour down the road, I noticed that the mattress pad on top of the trailer load kept lifting up and flapping. Several straps pulled loose. I pulled over and we spent another half hour re-securing the load. A long drive home. All of us were exhausted. Both Dave and Russ fell asleep. I tried to avoid any big bumps in the secondary roads we traveled.

Poor men. Early to bed tonight, I thought.

Dusk was settling in as I pulled into our driveway and drove around the house to the ramp. I limped a little as I stepped down and walked to Russ's door to help him get out. It took some maneuvering to get him, plus his walker and the oxygen tank, out of the car and up the ramp that leads to our back door. Dave already had the door unlocked and the dog out of the basement before Russ staggered into our kitchen. We made sure he was safely in a recliner before I went back to pull the car and trailer parallel to the deck for easier unloading. Dave was hungry so we waited until he ate a snack to tide him over. Then the two of us untied and unloaded Russ's bedsprings and mattress. I brought in a few other things, Russ's clothing, the folder from Hospice (to be turned over our local Hospice team tomorrow), and the cooler loaded with food and snacks from Russ's refrigerator in New York.

"The rest can wait until tomorrow, Dave."

He nodded and drove the car out front and backed it and the trailer into our garage for the night. We were all tired and cranky, but at last Russ was home, safe with us, and tomorrow was another day.

CHAPTER 19

Coping With Two Patients

The next day brought plenty of help. The nurses came first, assessed Russ, and signed him up for the program. They started reviewing our duties as caregivers, but I waved that away.

"Both Dave and I took care of my mother through Hospice," I said. "We remember the drill: in an emergency, don't call 911, call Hospice."

Next came the equipment truck. The driver was a wonderfully kind man who accidentally backed over Dave's tall flag pole. He came in the house, apologizing and actually weeping!

"I am so sorry, Mr. Bauer. I couldn't see your flag as I backed up."

Dave just grinned.

"No problem. It was just a plastic pole. I can put it up again later."

The guy brought a hospital bed, a table on wheels, a wheelchair, another walker (the Buffalo one had to be returned), and oxygen materials. This was a machine that took oxygen from the regular air in our house, condensed it, added moisture, and pumped it through the nasal canna for Russ's use. Best of all, the man set the machine up in our living room and taught me how to use everything. Dave watched but I realized the majority of the work would fall to me. Yesterday's moving fiasco left my husband drained of energy for several days.

Later that morning, a Hospice Chaplain arrived, and proceeded to help me finish unloading the trailer. A social worker also helped with that tiresome chore. Finally everyone left, and all three of us headed to our beds for a long autumn nap.

Supper time that night showed me just how weak Russ had become after battling cancer for so many months. He ate very little, took his pills with pudding, and retired back to bed. Thankfully, the hospital bed was adjustable so he could be propped up without struggling with pillows. We watched television until 9 p.m., then all of retired for the night. I made sure Russ had plenty of nightlights in case he needed to use the bathroom, just off our bedroom. I left the hallway door open for him, and kept our bedroom door closed to allow privacy. This sometimes proved a problem, since Dave often got up in the middle of the night to use the bathroom, too. Ended up with both doors to the bathroom open during the night, Dave insisted. Just a few of the many conflicts that arose as Russ's care created little problems in our household.

It took me a while to realize that my husband resented the time and effort I spent on our son's care. Formerly, all my care and attention centered on my husband's many medical needs. Now, suddenly, another man under our roof demanded just as much loving attention.

I can't believe this, I thought. *Suddenly I am torn between my husband and my son.*

Prayers to heaven during that time of adjustment consisted of pleas for patience. Recalling Jesus instructions to his disciples from Matthew's gospel, chapter 19, verse 30, about them being able to move mountains if they possessed even a small seed of faith, I prayed.

A mustard seed of patience, Lord, please.

Later this daily plea, added to the prayer petitions I recited after praying the Rosary, changed. I needed something bigger than a mustard seed of faith to deal with the daily frustrations of caring for two patients, both stubborn Bauer type men.

I need an avocado seed of patience, Lord, please?

Rather than confront my husband about his obvious jealousy, I ignored it. Really didn't want Russ to feel he was an unwanted guest in our home. Russ wasn't fooled. He complained to me.

"When you are busy in the kitchen, Mom. Dad won't even look at me."

I hated to take sides.

"Dad hasn't been the same since Jim died."

Russ looked away. "Yeah, I get it."

I felt guilty for not speaking to my husband about his sour moods. And I felt guilty because there wasn't enough of my time and energy to cover all my bases. I felt torn, inadequate, a failure as a caregiver.

What am I doing wrong, Lord? Dave is jealous and Russ feels rejected, unwanted in our home. Help!

This daily battle reminded me of Russ's childhood and how he must have felt when I raced past him without a glance, intent on taking care of all the details of running a household full of little people. A mother's guilt never seems to fade. I redoubled my efforts to keep peace in our so-called happy home.

Because Russ ate very little, and most of what he did enjoy was sweet and soft, I bought him his favorite treat, pudding, and added another sweet: ice cream sandwiches. Dave favored bowls of vanilla ice cream. He often loaded up his dish with huge amounts of that sweet treat and ate it in front of Russ without offering to share. Really, my jealous husband, as he slid further into Alzheimer's disease, was such a brat! I countered by sharing the ice cream sandwiches with Russ. An hour past supper, dishes done and dog walked, I would stand in the doorway between the living room and kitchen, holding an ice cream sandwich in each hand. One for each of us. I waved one at Russ and grinned. He always snapped-to and reached out for his nightly treat. I sat on the recliner beside his hospital bed, both of us enjoying our ice cream as we watched "Jeopardy " and "Wheel of Fortune" together. Thwarted at his own game, Dave snorted and retreated to the kitchen to work on his "Word Finder" puzzles.

Now, years later, I do not regret choosing to spend more time with my son than with my husband. Russ's time here on earth was very limited. Dave had my attention for over sixty years. We would survive his brief unseemly behavior, after we buried still another son.

CHAPTER 20

Russ's Final Days

Those days of Russ's too short life passed by in flurries of activity. Hospice nurses, doctor visits, the social worker coming (usually unannounced), a music therapist who charmed Russ with songs played on her guitar. Occasionally a sitter stayed with Russ when Dave had a doctor's appointment. Later, as our son's strength waned, a Bath Lady came to help Russ clean up. At first, Russ denied that he needed help taking a shower, and I believed him. I prepared clean clothing, towels and wash cloths, plus shampoo for his use. After putting the bath chair into the tub/shower, I helped Russ into the room and shut the door, giving him the privacy I thought he craved.

"Let me know when you are finished, Russ. I'll help you get back to bed."

It seemed only minutes later when he opened the door, fully dressed in clean pajamas, with his wet hair slicked down around his ears. It took me a while to realize the charade. Russ merely stuck his head under the running water, then pulled back and changed clothing. No soap. No shampoo. No real cleansing shower at all. From childhood on Russ hated water. I should have guessed sooner. *Crusty Rusty.*

More savvy than me about the ways of terminally ill patients, the visiting nurse soon insisted that a Bath Lady come to help out. I thought Russ would get stubborn about it, but he seemed to enjoy the extra attention of a friendly woman as they splashed behind closed doors.

I realized then that I might have cured Russ's aversion to bath time when he was a toddler. If I had bathed him alone, giving him plenty of splash time and extra attention, he may never have earned the nickname, Crusty Rusty. But Rusty was one of four toddlers, and I bathed them all together until they were old enough to be curious about the difference between male and female body parts. I have one old snapshot of the four of them in the tub. Davy, Cathy and Barb are all laughing and splashing. Rusty is hanging on the edge of the tub, looking absolutely miserable. Poor kid. I feel badly that I was such an unaware mother at that time.

Russ's strength waned visibly in the coming days. He went from using a walker, to full time use of the wheelchair. He needed help moving from bed to chair. I lacked the body strength to lift him. Dave did that chore with visible reluctance. It hurt me to see the two of them together. Russ so weak and helpless, Dave so rough and begrudging as he man-handled Russ into the waiting wheelchair. A glint of tears flashed in Russ's eyes. I brushed away my tears too.

Once in the chair, I wheeled Russ into the bathroom. I helped him as he grabbed the handle on the wall and maneuvered his body around so he could lower himself onto the toilet. Just before his bottom hit the seat, I would yank down his pajama bottom. It pained me to see his bony hips.

"Thanks Mom." he said with a long sigh.

"No problem, son. Call me when you are finished."

At first, I could move him from toilet to wheelchair again. But as Russ's arm strength vanished, we had to call Dad for help. Russ hated to depend on his father for help. Me too. At mealtime, the bed to wheelchair struggle had to be repeated. I wondered aloud if it might be easier on both guys if Russ ate his meals propped up in bed. Neither man liked my idea.

Dave gave me a scowl that meant, *Quit coddling the kid.*

Russ looked hurt. "Don't you want me to sit at the table with you, Mom?"

Lord, an avocado seed of patience, please?

So the bed to chair, and chair to bed dance continued.

Our sixtieth wedding anniversary approached. Hospice gave us the gift of extra time that day. Dave had an appointment at the Wound Center that morning. He suffered from seeping wounds on both legs, wounds that refused to close up and heal over. Being diabetic, the wounds were especially dangerous. Untreated, they could morph into major infection. I tried everything to cure those wounds, salves, pressure bandages, and an herbal remedy. Nothing worked. Our family doctor recommended the Wound Center.

Since Hospice gave us extra time that day, we planned to enjoy a nice lunch out. Unfortunately, the doctor's office was running behind that day. We waited an hour, an especially stressful hour, and still no beckoning invitation into the inner sanctum of the Wound Center office. Finally, I went to the desk and canceled the appointment.

"Our son is in Hospice," I said. She already knew this so it made me even angrier at the prolonged wait. "We need to go home. We'll have to reschedule."

Fuming, we left the building. No cozy anniversary luncheon celebration for us. We barely had time to hit Walmart for some food supplies before we raced home. The Hospice sitter was driving down our driveway as we pulled in. The next day, Thanksgiving, daughter Rose and her family came down for the day. They had planned a non-traditional meal for the holiday. Rose knew how busy and stressed we all were. I had neither strength nor inclination to fuss over a full turkey dinner.

"Mom? How about if we bring down a nice lasagna for supper?"

Bless her and her husband, Flo, the chef of their family!

"Thanks. Sounds wonderful."

Turned out that wonderful meal was actually Russ's last supper.

He sat beside me so I could help him with the food. We began with our usual Grace before meals, and Russ joined in, smiling. He leaned over to whisper.

"See, Mom? I remembered this time."

As the meal progressed, I noticed Russ was picking at the pasta with his fingers. He grabbed up pieces of lasagna and popped them into his mouth, like a toddler learning to eat people food. I leaned over, grabbed his sticky hand, wiped it off with a napkin, and pointed at his fork. Staring at me for a long moment, he finally took the hint and picked up his utensil. Sitting on the other side of Russ, Dad never lifted his head or noticed. When my Dave ate, he concentrated on his food! Sometimes that was a good thing.

We all ate well. Russ even had two pieces of pie, with Cool Whip piled on top like a snow cone. After doing all the meal clean up, and exchanging hugs all around, Rose and family left for home. It meant a long drive through darkness for them to return to their home in western New York, but they had wanted to spend Thanksgiving with us. Meant so much to me to have extended family together after struggling alone with the two guys I battled every day.

Just before bedtime, Russ needed the bathroom. I helped him, as I always did, settling him on the toilet before closing the door.

"Call me when you are finished."

Dave and I lingered by the kitchen sink as I put away a few

dishes left out by the clean-up crew. He reached to encircle me in one of his bear hugs. I snuggled against him, glad for this rare gesture of affection. Suddenly, I had to pull away.

"Did you hear that?"

Dave, even with his high tech hearing aids, did not hear very clearly most of the time.

"What?"

"I think Russ fell in the bathroom."

He lay helplessly prone on the thin carpet of the bathroom.

"Can you sit up, Russ?"

He struggled but could not get his arms to lift his body into an upright position.

"I'll get Dad."

"No!" But then he admitted how helpless he felt. "OK. Call Dad. I can't get up alone."

Even with Dave's manly strength, it took both of us to lift Russ into his wheelchair again. The chair to bed maneuver seemed especially difficult too. Russ fell against his pillows with a deep sigh. We were all sweating from the physical effort. Dave straightened up and rubbed his back, groaning. My back talked to me too, saying, *"Are you crazy? Lifting a dead weight like that? You're not young anymore, ya know!"*

As he lay there that evening, panting from the exertion of his bathroom trip and the resulting painful push/shove into bed, Russ turned slowly to me. I rested in my recliner, waiting for Dave to finish up in the bathroom so I could get ready for bed, too.

"Mom? Do you see that woman in a white dress standing at the foot of my bed?"

He pointed, but I saw nothing there. I shook my head. *Russ must be hallucinating.* Frowning, he heaved a long frustrated sigh.

"But I think I saw Jim's shadow in the kitchen a bit ago," I told him, truthfully.

I had noticed the barest shadow reflected in the glass of the china cabinet a few moments before. The shadow/vision looked like the profile of son Jim, his ever present ball cap, the scraggly beard he wore the last time I saw him alive.

Russ sat up straighter. His arms reached for me. I stood up to embrace him. He hugged me tightly, his face buried against my shoulder. This was such an unusual event for the both of us. Russ had never been the demonstrative type. I couldn't remember the last time we hugged like this. In fact, I believe this was the first time he had hugged me so warmly since childhood! I patted his back as he stifled a sob.

"Mom. I'm afraid of the end."

I rubbed his stiff shoulders, struggling to compose myself. Tears would not help my son now as he faced his future with fearful dread.

"It will be OK, Russ. You will just fall asleep when the time comes. No pain, thanks to those potent drugs you take. Then you will wake up in heaven and get to see your brothers again."

He sniffed. "You think so, Mom?"

"I know so, Russ. Davy and Jim are waiting for you. So are all your grandparents. Remember how Grandpa Ramier fussed over you? I think you were his favorite."

He heaved a long sigh and sank back against his pillows.

"Might be that lady in white I saw might be an angel, ya think, Mom?"

I nodded, unable to speak. Russ must have seen his guardian angel waiting to welcome him Home. He asked for extra pain medicine that night. He took strong pain pills four times a day. When he was really hurting, he asked for and received a half dropper of liquid morphine sulfate.

We all went to bed early that night.

CHAPTER 21

The Vigil

Next morning, Russ was not himself. He had used his urinal during the night, rather than try to make it to the bathroom. I emptied it without comment, grateful he had not attempted to move his frail body from bed to chair without help. Dave helped me put Russ in his chair for breakfast. Our son's body seemed especially limp as he slid off the side of the bed and plopped into the wheelchair. He asked for dry cereal and I poured it into a wide bowl, added milk, and handed him a spoon. His morning meds were already in a small cup beside his plate. He refused coffee. Dave sat across the table, reading the morning paper as he sipped his coffee.

Time to walk the dog. Morning dog walk belonged to me. I used the time outside to pray the rosary as Smokey loped along, pausing to sniff every twig and blade of grass. The dog loved being outside in the wilds of our country home. It was cool that morning, so we walked briskly, and returned home in less than a half hour.

"Nice and warm in here," I murmured as I peeled off winter garments. My hands and cheeks warmed quickly in the small laundry room off the back door as I pulled off my boots. The scene in the kitchen felt like a cold slap in the face. First thing I noticed was the expression of disgust on Dave's face. My husband pointed at Russ.

"Look at him! He lifted up his cereal bowl and poured milk all over his face, and down the front of his shirt."

My heart sank.

"And now he just sits there grinning. He won't even sit up straight."

I sat beside Russ, assessing him. Dave was right, Russ was slumped over to one side, his arm dangling over the side of his chair. I noticed his pill container had not been touched. I pulled our son upright in the chair, speaking quietly to him.

"Are you all right, Russ?"

No answer, just that silly grin.

I picked up the pills and poured them into my hand.

"These are your pain medications, Russ. Better take them."

His head rolled to one side as he stared up at me. He nodded. But when I tried to hand the pills to him, he could not grasp them. I leaned into the refrigerator and brought out a pudding cup. Taking his spoon, I buried a pill in the creamy dessert and spooned it into Russ's mouth.

He chewed the pill!

Horrified, I turned to Dave, who had been watching this little drama without commenting.

"I think Russ had a stroke, Dave. We need to put him to bed. Now!"

Easier said than done. It took every bit of strength Dave and I owned to lift our son out of the wheelchair and into his bed. Russ could not help in any way. He felt limp as a rag doll and fifty times as heavy as he did last night. When finally we managed to heft his body onto the edge of the bed his bony bottom still hung in mid air. Dave gave a final shove and Russ rolled into the center of the bed.

"Geez, Dad," Russ protested. "You crushed my balls!"

It was the last sentence our son ever uttered.

Hospice nurses came pretty quickly after I explained what happened. By that time, Russ was in a coma, spiking a fever, completely unresponsive. They hustled around his bed, stripping off his milk-wet clothing, washing him, and inserting a catheter. Several cups of urine gushed into the catch bag. He must have been holding it all in, not wanting to endure the physical stress of trying to use the bathroom.

The nurse brought new medication, all liquids. She left written instructions on dosage and times to give them. One medication was an anti-convulsive, the other a second bottle of morphine.

"If he seems to be in pain, don't be afraid to give these meds as often as he needs it to make him comfortable."

The anti-convulsive had a two hour dosage, the morphine, every hour, as needed.

"You don't have to stroke his throat to make him swallow it. Just lift his lip and squirt it into the side of his cheek. His mucus membranes will absorb it."

So our death vigil began. Russ had his stroke on Friday. His fever raged all weekend. He never woke up again. Sunday evening, November 25, 2012, he breathed his last.

It was past bedtime for me, 9:30 p.m. I decided to sleep in my recliner beside Russ's hospital bed, in case he cried out in pain during the night. As I yawned, Russ, who had been panting, gave one final gasp and stopped breathing. I waited a bit, thinking he would resume his tortured struggle to breathe. Quiet in the room, except for the oxygen machine pumping away. I stood up and stared at my son's lifeless body. His dark eyes were half open. No more panting breaths. I shook his shoulder a bit. No response. I grabbed a flashlight and shined it into those dark eyes. No blink, no widening nor narrowing of the pupils.

He's gone, Mom. The voice in my head sounded like Jim's.

With a small sound of grief, I hurried to our bedroom. Dave, undressing beside the bed, looked exhausted. His shoulders slumped as he untied his shoes.

"I think Russ died," I said, sinking down on the edge of the mattress.

Dave turned to me. A slight smile of relief lit his dark expression. I felt like slapping him.

Our son just died and you have the nerve to smile!

"Yeah?" he said, and stood up.

I uncurled my fist and looked away. We both returned to the death bed. Dave used the flashlight too. He put a hand over Russ's mouth, held it there a few moments, then shook his head.

"Poor kid. At least he's not suffering anymore," he said softly.

He reached over and gently closed our son's eyes.

My urge to slap him faded as I witnessed my husband's true self, the kind and gentle husband and father I had loved for over sixty years.

I could not cry.
How bitter do you risk becoming
by swallowing too many tears?

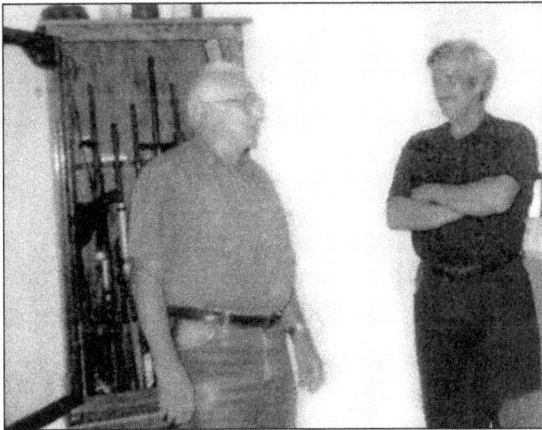

Daddy Dave and Russ

CHAPTER 22

Too Many Funerals

Russell died November 25, 2012, less than fifteen months after son Jim died, a few days short of two months after his oldest brother Davy passed away. Daddy Dave and I had lost three sons within such a short period of time. Neither of us seemed capable of mourning yet another loss. We were shell-shocked veterans of the death war. We stared at each other that evening, helpless, and numb. We hugged briefly, then I pulled away to make the phone calls. Greg Borland, the local mortician and a good friend, answered on the first ring. He had been waiting, alerted by an earlier message from us.

"Russ just died," I said.

"Poor guy. May he rest in peace," Greg said. "I'll be right over."

"I called the Hospice nurse and she should be here in about an hour," I told him and had to smile. "She is coming up from New Bethlehem. She said twenty minutes, but we both know it takes longer than that to drive up here."

"If you don't mind, I'll come now anyway. We can make a few plans. OK?"

"Sure, Greg. But I want the nurse to pronounce the death. Don't want any questions later from his son. Russ and his boy had a contentious relationship."

"I understand. See you in a bit."

Russ and his son, Tony, had forged a fragile truce in the days before we brought him home to Pennsylvania. As Russ grew weaker in his western New York house spending every day confined to his bed, Tony began to drop by occasionally. Later, he visited his biological father at least once a week, bringing pizza, and a listening ear. Neither man did a lot of talking, but his son just being there meant a lot to Russ. I know our son harbored deep regret for the way he had abandoned his only child. As his days here with us grew shorter, Russ asked Tony to come visit. I think he wanted to clear the air while he still had the chance. But Tony never came, even when I reminded him several times via email. Now it was too late.

True to his word, Greg arrived within fifteen minutes. His black hearse waited out front, the motor running to keep his assistant warm.

"It may be a while, Greg. Why not bring your helper inside? Warmer than in a cold vehicle."

Greg stepped away from our hug and grinned.

"The guy is new. He is a bit leery about intruding on a family's new grief."

We did make a few funeral plans as we all waited for the Hospice nurse. Greg jotted down a few statistics about Russ's life and family. We discussed day and time of Wake and funeral. Didn't need to name Russ's siblings. Greg still had the list from Jim's memorial funeral Mass last year. The only additional information needed was the death date of Dave Jr., and the name of Russ's son.

"I don't know whether Tony will come to his father's funeral, or not."

I heaved a long sigh, exhausted from the death vigil and the energy-sapping long days of worry and stress. Greg touched my arm.

"We can take care of the rest of this tomorrow, Cecile. Why don't you sit down now? Have a cup of coffee or a stiff drink?"

I shook my head.

"How about you, Dave? You look pretty worn out to me."

Dave nodded and sank into his recliner. He shook his head.

"I don't know how much more of this I can take," he muttered.

I found his favorite chair blanket and covered him up. He patted my hand and looked away. I noticed he fished for his handkerchief and took a long swipe at his nose. But I couldn't cry.

Why Lord? Why can't I cry for my loved ones? Am I so stone-hearted that another death in our family just leaves me cold and numb?

I didn't know the answer then. It took me long months before I came to terms with our family losses. Before I understood why I couldn't cry. Before God melted my frozen heart.

After the nurse arrived, flushed and full of apologies, she pronounced Russ's death and removed his catheter. Dave gathered up the tubing and the catch bag and dumped them outside in the burn barrel. He came inside, shivering.

"Must be zero out there," he said and rubbed his frozen hands together.

Greg's assistant entered the room, carrying a folded up gurney and a black body bag. The two men moved my recliner in order to position the gurney beside the hospital bed. Both men leaned across the narrow table trying to grab Russ's body to slide it over. The nurse tried to shield me but I brushed her away.

"I want to watch!" I snapped. She backed off.

"Greg, there is a draw sheet under Russ. Use that to slide him over."

He nodded and reached for the flowered sheet. As they slid the limp body of our son onto the table, his head lolled to the side. His beard, the long face marked with suffering, transformed into something mystical before my eyes.

I saw the face of Christ, just as his beloved mother must have viewed her crucified son as they lowered him down from the cross.

Now I could cry and I did.

CHAPTER 23

Lost in Leeper

The morning of Russ's funeral dawned sunny and bright. The family assembled the night before, and most stayed overnight. It had been a small Wake. No one in our parish knew our son Russ, but they came to comfort Dave and me just the same. Even our youngest son, Mike, came despite the fight the two brothers had months before and never resolved. He had called earlier in the week to offer sympathy. I told him we were desperate for pall bearers, and he offered to bring his grown son, Justin with him.

"Oh, thanks so much, Mike. I didn't know if you would come or not."

"He's still my brother, Mom."

The family was expected at the funeral home at nine a.m. for the closing prayers before lining up for the funeral procession to the church. It took several cars to ferry all the gathered family to Leeper. Dave and his sister, Betty, a nun, rode with me. All the way to the funeral home I fretted silently about daughter Cathy, driving down from Buffalo. Cathy is what I call direction-challenged. She can get lost in a parking lot. As I sailed through Leeper, worrying about Cathy, I passed the funeral home and kept on going. From the back seat, Sister Betty cleared her throat.

"Where are you headed? she asked.

Dave turned to stare at me. "You drove right past Borland's," he said.

"Oops," I said and turned around in the first driveway available.

When we drove into the parking lot at Borland's, Cathy waved and giggled. She stood right next to Greg, the mortician.

"I thought I was the only one who got lost driving," she said, grinning.

Greg said, "You know, Cecile, I never knew anyone who got lost in Leeper. Never."

"Well, now you do," I said and had to laugh.

Lost in Leeper. Another funny family story to add to our collection. I believe that it is this tradition of love and laughter that has helped sustain our family through good times, and especially through the bad times. We laugh, because we are not so good at crying.

When the funeral procession entered the parking lot at our church, St. Mary's at Crown, Tony and his wife Denise climbed out of their car. I hurried over to hug them both.

"Thanks so much for coming!"

Tony helped spread the white pall over his father's coffin. We proceeded, all the Bauer siblings and grandchildren, behind Russ's body to the front of the church. Our family sticks together through thick and thin. *Thanks, God!*

CHAPTER 24

Daddy Dave's Long Struggle

After the deaths of our three sons, life never did resume in any normal fashion. We were changed, all of us, and Dave Sr. seemed changed the most of any of us.

Of course, his decline into dementia had already begun before our baby boy died. I remember the celebration of his 80th birthday at the park in western NY, and how prickly my husband seemed that day. It started off here at home, when I insisted on doing the driving. My husband's driving skills had deteriorated so much that I no longer trusted him behind the wheel.

When we arrived at the park, Dave headed to the men's restroom. When riled up for any reason (he resented me driving instead of him), his stomach gave him fits. That day, he suffered explosive bouts of diarrhea. He did a lot of pouting that day. He ate the delicious food, lovingly provided by his adult children and grandchildren, with a sour expression on his face. Most of the party goers steered clear of the guest of honor, pausing only long enough to give him a brief hug, and a loving greeting. One long glance at his mulish face and they backed away and returned to other family members, other relatives who were actually enjoying the day.

I did manage to snap one picture of Daddy Dave with son Jim and grandsons Jon and Bryan. Bryan did not want to be included in the group shot, but I caught the edge of his face nonetheless. The picture shows Daddy Dave as he slumps over a picnic table, face long and grouchy as chews a hot dog. Jon is half smiling, his hand on Grandpa's shoulder. Jim, eyes swollen with illness, is barely smiling. Later, his sisters remarked that Jim did not look well that day. I had noticed that Jim was keeping away from the rest of the family, eating alone on a back table. I went to sit with him, but he shooed me away.

"Better not sit with me, Mom. I'm just getting over the flu."

It was not flu, but alcoholic hepatitis, that made our youngest son so ill.

Fifty-five days later, Jim died.

CHAPTER 25

Dave's Health Issues

Dave's health became a problem shortly after we moved to Pennsylvania. Building our house had taken its toll on his strength. It did not help that he slipped and fell while moving a bundle of shingles from the porch roof to my waiting arms below. We used a rope method. He tied a bundle with a clothesline rope, then lowered it down to me, one bundle at a time. The last bundle stuck, frozen to the roof. Dave struggled to break it loose, and ended up falling onto his right side. Arm straight out to break his fall, he winced as the weight of his body twisted his shoulder. He climbed down the ladder slowly, favoring his arm, cussing at the pain.

"Now what are we going to do?" he said, his face twisted in frustration.

It was the day before Thanksgiving, 1995. Twice we had to shovel off the plywood cover on the roof in order to lay shingles. It had not been a good week at all. We were both feeling pressured to get the house "under cover" so we could move in. We had overstayed our welcome at Dave's brother's house. Like homeless relatives, barely tolerated as unwelcome guests, we *needed* to move into our own place.

Dave rubbed his injured shoulder and puffed with pain.

"How can I finish the back roof now?" he wailed. "My arm is useless!"

"Butch said he will finish the roof for us," I said.

Our nephew had been a God-send during the long process of building our home. We paid him whatever he asked, but I know he did not keep track of his actual hours, nor over-charge us for anything.

"We can't afford to pay anyone now," Dave said. "We're already over budget."

He threw down his tools and stomped away, his shoulders slumped in defeat.

I called after him.

"Dave! We can't afford *not* to pay someone right now. We need to move in!"

He threw up his hands, a familiar signal that he was ready to give up completely.

The day after Thanksgiving Butch, his brother Tony, and other men came to finish the back roof. Daughter Rose and family had arrived the day before and we enjoyed a wonderful Thanksgiving dinner, courtesy of Rose and family. Flo had also made a lasagna to be served to the workers on Friday, as they worked on the roof. I laid the pan on top of a kerosene heater brother Paul had given us. It sat in our bare bones kitchen, and warmed up that room, plus part of the living room. We had heat, food and coffee. We had men putting on the last of our roof.

God is good. God is Great. Thank you, God!

Dave watched from the back yard, frowning as the younger men scampered around the steep roof, laying shingles and chattering as they teased each other. Tony took a slide down the roof and almost fell the twenty feet to the ground, but caught himself in time. He stood up at the edge of the roof and laughed.

"Whee, what a ride!" He said and climbed back to help Butch attach the shingles.

Down cellar, brother Cyril, our reluctant host, and his son-in-law Randy set up the furnace. We were not the only Bauer relatives anxious to help us move into our own home. At noon, the roof was finished. The men came down, put away their tools, and stomped into our kitchen. They all raved over the tasty lasagna.

Two weeks later, we moved into our little house in the woods.

Thank you God, for willing workers and good generous people.
We were blessed indeed.

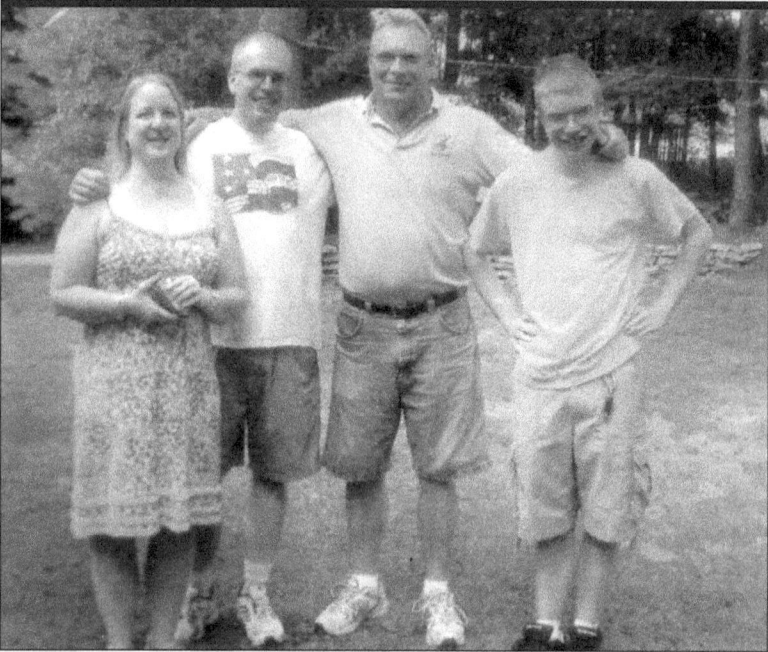

(L to R) Rose, Larry, Flo, and Dan

CHAPTER 26

In Our Own Home at Last

We moved into our unfinished camp-o-rama in the woods mid-December,1995. All winter we worked together installing drywall, putting up ceilings, painting, tiling, converting our house from a rough shell to a real country home. In the spring, we installed the vinyl siding, and built a deck out back, plus a long porch across the front of the house. The following year, we built a three-car garage. During those busy productive years, Dave's strength continued to be strong and healthy, although he did get tired more easily. I did too as we both grew older.

The winter of 1998, Dave's health began a steep decline. His energy fell, he was short of breath. An angioplasty revealed a serious heart defect. He needed open heart surgery and a valve replacement. Three years later, he had a second surgery to install a pacemaker. Those long years of hard work had taken a toll on my honey. He tired easily, became forgetful, dropped off to sleep as soon as he sat down no matter where he might be. That included the bathroom, the living room, the kitchen table, even at church. One Sunday, he fell asleep standing up! I pulled on his hand to ease him back onto the pew. Our family doctor did some tests, and put him on Aricept, an Alzheimer's medicine. Later she added a second medicine to his regimen, Namenda. He functioned almost normally, but our family noticed the difference.

"What's with Dad," they asked.

"Is he mad at us? He doesn't talk to us anymore."

True enough. Dave did seem mad at everyone. His hearing aids did not help him hear the clamorous conversations that marked any gathering of our large and noisy family. Unable to hear what the gang was laughing about, he decided they were all making fun of him. He stopped talking or trying to listen. Sleep was his escape, and he often escaped in the middle of any conversation. After we suffered the loss of our sons, Dave stopped trying to relate, to anyone, even me.

I told our family, "Dad hasn't been the same since Jim died."

But truly, he hadn't been himself for years before the deaths began.

CHAPTER 27

A Happy Event

One bright spot in our family occurred the summer of 2012. Mike's daughter Stephanie married her collage sweetheart Christopher.

As soon as we received the invitation, I began to fret about whether we should attend the celebration or not. It seems strange to me now, years after that troubled time in our lives, that I dreaded the thought of going to my beautiful granddaughter's wedding. It had been less than a year since we lost our youngest son. Still racked with grief and guilt over his untimely death, maybe I felt unworthy to celebrate anything? Grief takes many forms. Perhaps I was punishing myself by refusing to even consider enjoying myself in any way, especially a joyous occasion like a family wedding.

Then one Sunday, as I pulled Jim's cross necklace over my head, lips quivering as I remembered giving it to him for his 42nd birthday, I heard Jim's voice in my ears.

"Geez Mom, get a life!"

Only Jim would have the nerve to call me out like that! I grinned and dried my tears. Suddenly, I couldn't wait to go to Stephanie's wedding.

Thanks Jim for you irreverent, commonsense voice in my ears.

The wedding was well worth the effort it took to drive up to Niagara Falls, New York, to attend it. Barb, her husband Henry, and our son Jason from Arizona, plus Dave and I, filled Barb's rented car. Henry asked if we wanted to use our vehicle, a roomier SUV for the trip, but I explained why it did not seem like a good idea.

"If we take our car, Dad will want to drive. If we take your vehicle, you can drive and he won't pitch a fit about being a passenger."

Henry nodded. "I might need another driver later if I get too tired," he said.

"No problem, Henry. I can drive home, and we will spring for gas money too."

The wedding was beautiful and we all enjoyed ourselves. One unforgettable moment came when Mike, father of the bride, danced with his beautiful daughter. Everyone rushed to take pictures because Mike had tears in his eyes. This was a rare event for our tough, throw his glasses at the wall, second youngest son. The only other time I saw the adult Mike crying was after Jim's funeral, when he leaned into the car door to say goodbye to us before we drove home.

Several other photos show happy family members before and after the event. Davy and Bonnie were there and I treasure the pictures of them dressed up and looking so happy. Two months later, we lost Davy. This happy occasion was like an oasis in our grieving time. I am so grateful we attended the wedding.

We left the reception around ten, then started the long haul home. We stopped just south of Buffalo for gas. I handed Dave a couple of twenties to pay for gas and a round of sodas. While the guys were out of the car, I climbed out of the back seat and into the driver's seat. No one complained about this. Henry did ask, quite seriously, "Do you know the way home pretty good?"

I nodded, hiding a grin. I could have told Henry I had been making the Buffalo to Pennsylvania trip since I was an infant, but kept quiet about it. I could drive that route on auto pilot, and did that night. A few times I drifted off the edge of the road, hitting the rumble bars, but none of the passengers woke up from the vibrations. We arrived safely home at 3 a.m.

Thank you Lord for watching over our family. And thank you for the good memories of our granddaughter's wedding. It will sustain us for the uncertain future.

"You changed my mourning into dancing;
O LORD, my God,
forever will I give you thanks."
Psalms 30:12,13

CHAPTER 28

A Year of Healing

After the family wedding, the autumn months dragged past. I lost myself in computer games. Dave rode his lawn mower in endless circles as he cut any grass he could find to trim. We endured the deaths of two more sons, Davy and Russ, then settled in to survive the long snowy winter. When the snows came, Dave hooked up the plow to his ATV and kept the driveway and lane road open.

Spring came and the grass did not grow fast enough to keep Dave occupied. One day he decided to repair a ceiling light in the garage. He used an aluminum extension ladder to reach above the vehicles and work on the tube light. After I walked the dog that morning, Smokey and I went upstairs to my former writing workroom. It was my office in name only. I had no heart to write anything other than emails or to answer a post on Facebook.

A few hours later, engrossed in a game of Spider Solitaire, I missed the absence of sounds coming from the garage. No more hammering. Nor did I hear the portable drill. Suddenly, the dog rose up on his hind legs and stared out the window. His long nose pointed toward the open garage door. He whined. I tore my eyes away from the computer screen and glanced outside.

"I don't see anything, Smokey, " I said, petting the dog.

He whined again.

Moments later, the front door opened, and Dave stumbled into the living room. I should have realized something was very wrong, because Dave never came into the house that way. He always used the back door, hitting the adjoining bathroom first before entering the kitchen. I glanced at the clock, 10 a.m. Too early for lunch.

Now what? I thought and turned off the computer. Smokey raced down the steps.

Moments later I joined the dog and Dave in the living room. My husband sat on the couch, his head leaning against the backrest. His face looked gray. My first thought: *sugar dive.* I hurried to fetch the glucose tabs we kept for times when his diabetes acted up. I also grabbed a sport drink out of the fridge in case he was dehydrated. He accepted the sugar pills and took a sip from the bottled drink. I noticed his eyes looked weird. My brown-eyed honey now had the uncertain blue colored eyes of a newborn baby. I leaned forward for a closer look at his face.

Something is wrong.

"What happened, Dave?"

His strangely glazed eyes shifted to meet my stare. He shrugged and heaved a long sigh.

"I just took a two hour nap on the garage floor."

"What?"

"I don't know what happened. Last thing I remember is leaning against the car door, with the light fixture in my hands. Then I woke up on the cardboard."

Dave meant the large sheets of cardboard he spread on the garage floor to catch oil drips from the lawn mower and ATV. His hearing aids were missing. Later I found them side by side on the cardboard. He must have fallen from the ladder, and landed so hard the aids flew out of his ears when his head hit the floor. I called the ambulance, and for once, Dave didn't object.

At Clarion Hospital an x-ray showed a fractured skull with bleeding on the brain. A helicopter flew him to St. Vincent's Hospital in Erie.

For sixteen days, Dave stayed in the hospital while his brain bleed healed (without surgery, thank God!). He did physical therapy which he thoroughly enjoyed. All those kind nurses fussing over him, their words of praise as he gained strength, kept him busy and happy. Strange things happened, though. His day nurses loved him. His night nurses complained that he was a tough patient to control. Daughter Rose and I visited Dave every other day. His primary doctor at the hospital talked to us about Dave's conflicting reports.

"Why do you think Dave acts out at night but not during the day?" he asked us.

Rose shrugged. I sighed.

"I hope you have it on Dave's chart that he has Alzheimer's?"

"Yes, but …"

The doctor was puzzled and so were we. Later we discovered the evening nurse gave Dave an opiate-based sedative every evening to "settle him down for the night."

"Dave can't handle opiates," I protested. "They make him loopy. When he had his open heart surgery he managed to hold the sixth floor of St. Francis' hospital hostage before a doctor managed to talk him down."

The skeptical glance of the Erie doctor made me mad.

"Check his records. It should be on his chart! I told enough doctors and nurses about it!"

Despite my protests, the nurses continued to "sedate" Dave every evening. Dave continued to give them a hard time every night. All concerned were happy to see Dave leave for home after sixteen days. The discharge nurse slipped Dave a dose of the forbidden sedative before the trip.

Halfway home Dave's tirade began. He had a lot of grudges to air, most of them concerned the evening nurses, and how he never managed to get a good night's sleep. For miles, his rambling complaints went on and on. Finally I held up one hand.

"Dave, stop. I know you had a rough time at the hospital, but we are going home now. Can't you forget the bad times? It's a holiday weekend. Family is coming. Be happy!"

Dave settled into a sullen silence. Arms crossed, he stared out the window the rest of the way home. As I pulled the car around the back, he awoke from a doze and glanced around.

"Finally!" he said.

He opened his door and put one leg outside. But then he refused to get out of the car.

I hurried to unlock and open the back door in case Dave felt woozy walking in.

He refused to get out of the car.

"What? Do you need a hand?"

No answer. He stared straight ahead, mute as a mule. He refused my offered hand. I stared at his face. *What on earth is going on?* I tried everything to move him but he ignored my pleas. Finally I retreated, weeping, to sit on the deck and howl.

"Why are you acting like this? Do I need to drive you back to the hospital?"

He glared at me.

"Why don't you just take me out behind the garage and shoot me?"

"Don't tempt me!"

Finally, as the opiate drug wore off, and our visiting family members arrived, Dave consented to climb out of the car and enter the house. He smiled and hugged everyone, except me, of course. I was his enemy of the day.

But reason won out over strange reactions to forbidden drugs and life went on.

Thank you God.

CHAPTER 29

The Quack

During the winter of 2012, Dave's health problems increased. He spent a lot of time in the bathroom, falling asleep while leaning against the wall. Dave had always been a modest man, guarding against any accidental nakedness with the fierceness of an old nun. If I dared open the bathroom door to check on him, his outraged glare warned me away. Finally one day, I risked an argument to ask him about it.

"Is everything all right with you? You spend a lot of time in the bathroom these days."

He flushed and glanced away from my steady stare. After a long pause, when he realized I wouldn't just drop it this time, he answered.

"Something is haywire with my water system."

He bit his lip.

"Oh?" I waited for more information.

He blushed.

"Sometimes I can't pee. Other times I don't make it into the bathroom in time."

"So, you have a little dribble now and then?"

"More often these days."

"How long has this been happening to you?"

"Oh, maybe six months or so," he said, embarrassed.

We were sitting side by side at the supper table. I put my arm around his shoulder and leaned closer for a hug.

"I read somewhere that this happens to men your age. Tomorrow I'll call and make an appointment with our doctor."

He gave one of his famous hugs.

"Thanks, Hon. I didn't know how to tell you about it."

Our family doctor gave Dave a thorough exam, including the "assume the position" probe. She glanced at me, puzzled.

"I don't feel any growth inside. Maybe you better see a specialist to rule out a prostate problem."

Thus began our sad saga with the quack doctor I will label Doctor A. The urologist, Dr. A had a thick accent. I could understand him but he talked too quickly for Dave to comprehend his directions. As usual, when we were in a new doctor's office, I did the translating for Dave and also did most of the answering to the doctor's questions. Dave's head swivelled back and forth, his eyes puzzled, at the quick exchange between us.

Finally, Dr. A blurted, "Does he speak?"

I bristled at his rude tone of voice.

"Of course Dave speaks. He just doesn't hear very well. Your speech is tough to understand, even for me. And I have perfect hearing."

Dr. A glanced at his assistant and rolled his eyes. After that, the doc aimed his remarks at me. After a quick internal exam, he frowned, and peeled off his glove.

"Tell him to empty his bladder."

Moments later, Dave came back and climbed onto the exam table for an ultrasound of his lower abdomen. Neither Dave nor I appreciated the rude way Dr. A shoved Dave's garments down until his private area was fully exposed. I bit my tongue. If I made a scene about the intrusion on Dave's modesty, he might have gone into a rage and left the exam room in full dragon mode. The doctor tapped on the monitor screen and spoke to the assistant.

"See this? He can't empty his bladder completely. I felt two growths before. He needs a biopsy, the sooner the better."

We were ushered into another room with a secretary. She took down Dave's health history. Studying her laptop, she gave us an appointment for Dave's surgery in two weeks. She printed out a few sheets of pre-op instructions and handed them to me. I scanned the first few paragraphs then held up an instruction sheet and tapped on it.

"This says Dave needs to go off his blood thinner for two weeks before his biopsy."

I shook my head.

"Dave has an artificial heart valve. He needs his blood thinner to avoid a fatal blood clot."

She frowned. "Doctor insists patients go off blood thinners before he will operate."

"Well then, I guess you will have to cancel the biopsy."

"You have no right to make that decision," she huffed.

"I am my husband's health proxy, and he *will not* go two weeks without his blood thinner."

I stood up, ready to leave. The secretary backed off.

"Tell you what, Mrs. Bauer. Let me run this past Dr. A and your family doctor before we make any hasty decisions."

"Don't forget to talk to his heart doctor, too," I said and pointed to that doctor's phone number listed on Dave's health sheet. Dave stood at my elbow. We both turned to leave.

"I'll call you later," she said, as we walked away.

"What was that all about?" Dave said as we rode down the elevator. He grinned. "You looked pretty mad about something."

I explained about the pre-op instructions. His eyes widened when I mentioned the two week rule about blood thinners.

"What? Are they trying to kill me?" He shook his head in disgust. "I just don't trust a doctor that won't talk plainly to me."

I felt the same way, in spades. I should have followed my gut feeling and refused to allow Dave to undergo a biopsy with a doctor neither of us trusted. But the specter of prostate cancer reared its ugly head to frighten both of us.

After a conference call with Dave's three doctors, a compromise was reached. Three days without blood thinners. The first scheduled day off the thinner was a Sunday. I gave Dave his thinner that day anyhow. Two days seemed risky enough for him to be without this vital medicine.

Monday morning, a nurse from the heart doctor in Erie called me.

"Mrs. Bauer. I am so sorry, but there was a mix-up about Dave's medicine schedule. He needs to go to the Clarion hospital now and be put on special medicine before his biopsy tomorrow. He is already registered there."

"Great! Dave is going to love this," I said. "He hates even the idea of going into any hospital. Then to go a day early and stay overnight?" I sighed. "What happened to make the heart doctor change his mind?"

The nurse cleared her throat, embarrassed.

"When we had the three-way conference call, it was doctor's assistant who made that decision. He didn't read all of Mr. Bauer's chart."

"You mean the part about his artificial heart valve?"

I groaned, dreading the near future when I would need to persuade Dave to enter the hospital a day early. Leaving right now was out of the question. We would have lunch first. I know how hospitals are: no regard for a patient with diabetes who needs to eat at regular times. The nurse apologized again before urging me to drive Dave to the hospital immediately. I didn't tell her he had taken his blood thinner the evening before. They screwed up. Let them stew about it until we had a peaceful lunch. The long years of being my husband's health proxy made me tough and sometimes downright rude to nurses, doctors, and any health care professional who dared to put my hubby's health at risk with their mistakes.

The next morning Dave underwent the biopsy. Doctor A found and removed two growths from Dave's prostate gland. The procedure left Dave sore and bleeding. He needed to wear a pad to keep from staining his clothing. His urine drip continued, more often now that his organs had been roughly treated. He was not a happy camper.

After his biopsy showed two growths, I decided to call Dave's health insurance company in New York. After retiring from the New York State Thruway, his health coverage continued. It included the availability of Roswell Park Cancer Center of Excellence in Buffalo New York. This is a world renowned cancer treatment center. I made an appointment for March 1st.

Meanwhile, Dave had a follow up appointment with Dr. A. It did not go well. We sat in a small room. The doctor hid behind his desk with his laptop open, the screen facing away from us. As soon as we were seated the doctor shook his head. He did not look toward Dave but directed his remarks to me, as if Dave were a dumb animal, unable to understand what was happening.

"The biopsy report shows cancer," he said bluntly and leaned back waiting for my reaction.

I had been expecting the bad news.

"So, what's next? Surgery? Radiation seeds?"

He shook his head and spread his hands.

"I can do nothing for him. He's just an old man with a bad heart. He would die on the table."

For the first time in a long time, I was really glad Dave did not hear well. I should have asked, "So why did you perform the biopsy in the first place if he is too old for treatment?" But fear stalled my rational thinking. Instead, I said, "There must be something you can do!"

Doctor leaned forward.

"I can give him a hormone shot," he offered. "Might slow the growth of the cancer a bit."

Dave suffered the painful shot without complaint. Later this quack doctor had the nerve to send a bill to Medicare for *chemotherapy* for what he labeled a hormone shot!

I waited until we were home before I told Dave what the doctor has said about him being an old man. Dave stood up and shook his fist.

"You should have told me what he said. I would have reached across the desk and showed him who was a sick old man!"

I grinned. "That's why I didn't tell you at the time."

We hugged, clinging to each other. The specter of cancer hung heavy over our hearts. A multitude of our loved ones had succumbed to that dread disease already. My mother and sister, Dave's nephew Butch and niece Trudy, and more than a dozen of my first cousins, all died fighting cancer. I dreaded to even contemplate Dave suffering a painful death from cancer. *He wouldn't even be able to find relief in powerful pain medications,* I thought. Fear gripped my heart.

Dave had a really bad reaction to Percocet and Darvocet, opiate pain medications while recovering from his open heart surgery in 1998. He had gone loony-tunes in his hospital room.

I thought about this now as Dave and I clung together.

What would happen when Dave's cancer grows? How would I keep him comfortable in his last days of acute suffering? O God, please save Dave this agony. Wrap him in your loving arms, O Savior of the world. Guide the doctors at Roswell with your wisdom and power.

I gave Dave an extra warm hug.

"Lot's of fight left in you, Honey. We'll see what the doctors at Roswell say about your chances to beat this thing."

CHAPTER 30

The Miracle of Roswell

March 1st, we left early to drive up to Buffalo. Our appointment was for 1 p.m. We allowed plenty of time to get lost a few times in the city. It had been years since we drove in downtown Buffalo. Traffic patterns had changed considerably. Of course we took the wrong exit off the Skyway bridge, and then circled back to the Main Street exit.

"People in the city drive crazy!"

Dave yelped as another car pulled out in front of us. Fortunately, we managed to avoid collisions and found the correct street leading to the famous Cancer Center. I pulled out the cooler, the sandwiches, and Dave's pill bottle. We ate slowly, both of us dreading what lay ahead. The future looked dark and frightening at that moment in time. We munched on our sandwiches, stalling as long as we dared. Finally, we went inside to discover Dave's uncertain fate.

As soon as we entered the large foyer, the sound of music met us. Someone played a grand piano. The music sounded peaceful and welcoming as it echoed down the long hallway leading to

Patient Admissions. I stepped up to the first desk we came to, handing the worker Dave's appointment paper. We must have looked suspicious as we entered the building because I had noticed a security guard dogging our heels. As soon as the worker smiled and nodded at us, the guard faded away.

"Welcome to Roswell," the clerk said. She pointed to a nearby group of chairs. "Someone will be with you in a few minutes."

We sat down and took off our winter coats.

Soon a young man approached us. "Mr. Bauer?"

We both nodded. He extended his hand to Dave and nodded at me.

"I am John Brown, your health advocate. I will be with you the entire time you are here today. Welcome."

He escorted us to a nearby window. The clerk behind the counter took our paperwork, which included the DVD taken during Dave's biopsy. We filled out a few forms and were handed a blue card, Dave's official health card for Roswell Cancer Center in case he needed to come back for treatment. Mr. Brown explained all the benefits we were given while under the Roswell umbrella. There were suites we could stay in overnight or weekly, if needed, at no charge. Our travel expenses, mileage (we traveled 280 miles round trip) and meals would be reimbursed. All this wonderful care, explained in the warm accepting atmosphere, made me dizzy with relief.

At last, Dave is in the right place for the best of care. Thank you, God.

Mr. Brown stayed with us as Dave entered several rooms for exams. Within a half hour, we were escorted to a conference room with a large oak table surrounded by comfortable chairs. As we waited for the doctors to assemble, I leaned close to Dave and whispered.

"This is the royal treatment, Dave. I could get used to this."

It made him smile and relax. Mission accomplished. Mr. Brown nodded and smiled.

As soon as the main doctor, Doctor H (for hope), sat down, he frowned.

"Mr. Bauer. Why did your urologist even order a biopsy?"

He tapped the DVD case in his hand. Doctor H, the head urologist/oncology specialist appeared disgusted. My heart sank. Dave just stared at him. Our health advocate spoke up.

"Is there a problem, Doctor?" His voice held a warning.

"No, no problem. I guess that is the problem," he said and smiled.

He tapped a sheet of paper.

"Look here, Mr. Bauer."

We both leaned forward to examine a graph with numbers and statistics, which might as well have been written in Greek for all we understood about them. Mr. Brown read the graph too. Then he smiled and leaned back.

"It's good news, folks. Mr. Bauer, this is a wonderful report."

We were mystified as we glanced from the doctors to our advocate.

Dr. H smiled again.

"Mr. Bauer, your growths appeared to be so small and so slow growing that you will die of old age before you ever have to worry about cancer."

Dave blurted. "But that other doctor in Clarion told us I was too old for treatment."

I chimed in.

"Dr. A said Dave was just an old man with a bad heart and he would probably die on the operating table."

The cancer specialist's face darkened. He leaned forward and scowled.

"That doctor is a quack! And if he dares to send you a bill, don't pay it!"

Dave and I thanked all the men in the room. Our hearts were light indeed as we skipped down the hallway. At the reception area, a different musician was playing a guitar and singing, "Blowing in the Wind." If I ever get cancer, I will have nothing to fear as long as Roswell Park Cancer Center continues to exist.

Thank you God, for saving Dave from cancer. And thank you for doctors who genuinely practice good medicine.

Best of all, Dr. H (for hope) reported Dr. A to Medicare, and they denied his claim for payment. Later this quack packed up and left our area. Family suggested we sue for malpractice, for the needless pain and suffering he put Dave through. But we feared Dave's other doctors, our family doctor and his heart doctor, might be swept up in a class action suit. Money is not our God. We let the matter drop, satisfied when Dr. A quit his practice and moved away.

Lesson learned: if a doctor raises any uncertainty or suspicion in your heart, time to leave. In fact, run for the hills. Save yourself and your loved ones from the torture and pain that my honey suffered at the hands of the Quack.

CHAPTER 31

Dave Fades

As Dave recovered from his "treatment" for prostate cancer, his mental health seemed to decline more rapidly. He spent hours staring out the window, often dozing in his recliner, sleeping the long hours away. A previously strong farmer boy since his youth, now his aging body lost strength every day. His turn at dog walking became shorter and shorter. Where he had once strolled for most of an hour, enjoying the fresh air as our dog roamed over fields and woods, now Dave barely walked a thousand feet before returning to sit on the back deck. If I asked him if he felt all right, he would shrug and avoid my glance. He liked to stare into the sky, as leaves tumbled from our numerous oak and maple trees.

What did he see in those mild blue skies? Did he fear dying, worried about what awaited him in the next world? I never asked him about it and he did not volunteer any insight into his silent faith life. Yet ever the farm boy, he did not linger long on the back deck.

"Wasting time," he said. "Leaves are piling up."

He slapped his knees, stood up, and went to the garage to hook up the garden trailer.

One day that long autumn, as I prepared supper, Dave did not appear at the back door. He had a pretty accurate stomach timed exactly to the hours we sat down to eat. Four o'clock meant supper time. He never missed it. I went out the back door. No tractor noise. No Dave either. I circled the house calling his name. Suddenly I spotted a plaid shirt prone on the front lawn beneath the apple trees.

"Oh, no!"

Dave lay on his stomach, plucking at weeds in the grass. He glanced up as I raced to him.

"Are you OK?

He nodded and laughed a little.

"I just can't get up. Tried a couple of times, but kept losing my balance." He shrugged and rolled onto his back to look up at me. "Kinda dizzy today."

He held out his hand. I tried, but could not lift him.

"Should I call Randy (our nephew) to come and help?"

He scowled. "No! I'm not helpless. Just bring me my cane."

I raced for his cane. Between the cane and Dave leaning on me, we managed to get him back into the house. He collapsed onto his chair at the table.

"Whew! Thought I might miss supper tonight," he said and grinned faintly.

Dave's dizzy spells continued. Our doctor diagnosed a middle ear problem. Dave refused to take Antivert for it.

"I take too many pills now!" he protested.

Doctor turned to me. "Keep an eye on him."

I nodded. "Already do. Every day, a new surprise."

She gave me a sympathetic glance and patted my hand.

Another day Dave did not return from his evening dog walk. I waited, watching the clock, as I washed up the dishes.

Finally I noticed our pup, Smokey, sitting at the top of our property at the edge of the corn field. I walked out on the deck and called the dog. He refused to come. Smokey kept staring behind him, pawing the grass, whining. I called him again. No response.

Uh oh!

I flew down the steps and headed up to the field. Dave stood 1000 feet away, hanging onto the limb of a strong bush, weaving and unsteady on his feet.

"What happened? Are you OK?"

He looked embarrassed.

"Think I walked too far today. Legs won't go any farther."

I tried helping him, urging him to lean of me on one side while he used his cane for balance. We could not match our steps and Dave almost tumbled to the ground. He managed to grab another branch to steady himself. I took out my cell phone.

"What are you doing? You better not call an ambulance!"

"No. I'm calling Randy. If he's not home, I'll call one of our neighbor's sons to come help."

"Oh for Pete's sake! I could crawl home before anyone got here."

I shook my head. "It's either Randy, or I call 911. Take your pick."

He muttered a curse and shook his head. Not waiting for his decision, I speed dialed our nephew who lives a mile away. Randy picked up on the first ring and came within minutes. Meanwhile I ran back to our campfire area and grabbed up a lawn chair so Dave could sit down and rest.

Randy knew exactly what to do. Trained to be an EMT, he slowly walked Dave toward our house step by step. Take five steps, stop and rest. While supporting Dave with one long arm (Randy is a big man and he towered over Dave), our nephew kept up an ongoing conversation with my staggering husband. Randy walked

Dave up the ramp he had built for us, through the back door and on to his recliner in the living room. Dave collapsed into his chair with a long sigh.

"Thanks," he whispered. "For a while there I didn't think I would ever get home again."

Randy stood watching Dave for several minutes. Finally he glanced at me.

"Aunt C? You have a beer for me?"

I nodded and fetched him a cold can. I knew, without asking, that Randy wanted to extend his visit for a while in order to watch Dave for further evidence of a stroke.

I brought a sport drink for Dave. He sipped slowly, then put it aside. Randy nursed his beer until dark, then left, satisfied that Dave had just over-extended his energy and not suffered a stroke. He stopped at the door to remind me.

"Keep an eye on him, OK, Aunt C?"

I nodded and gave him a long hug.

"That's my job. Thanks for coming Randy."

Thank God for willing helpers, and thank God for Randy.

CHAPTER 32

After the Funerals

That autumn of 2013, life seemed to slow down even more. Dave's lawn chores were finished for the year. No more leaves to rake nor grass to cut. He did a lot of sleeping by the window, our dog snuggled beside his chair keeping watch on his master. I played computer games and visited Facebook for family news. Occasionally, something funny on the social network prompted me to drag Dave upstairs to watch something on U-Tube. He groaned as he climbed the steps to my computer room. His bones ached, he often complained.

"I just don't feel like doing anything," he moaned.

I knew that blah feeling, too. Somehow, since we began losing our sons to death, my avocation to write anything worthwhile had faded. My work computer sat idle, covered with a long beach towel. *Will I ever write again?* I wondered. At that point in time, I didn't even care.

One evening, going through collected paperwork on the desk near Dave's recliner, I found two magazines. They were "Word Finder" books, part of a collection Russ brought with him from

New York. I offered them to Dave. He shrugged and closed his eyes, ready for another nap. I took them to the kitchen table and laid them beside Dave's place mat, hoping he might get interested in the puzzles later. A few days later, Dave opened one of the magazines, thumbing through the pages with mild interest. He picked up a pen and circled a word that jumped out at him. Soon those word puzzles became an abiding interest for Dave. He poured over the words anytime he sat at the kitchen table. Soon he stayed at the table after supper and long into the evening. Television programs that had been his favorites no longer caught his interest. Several times he frowned as commercials came on.

"Do you understand what is going on?" he said, pointing to the television screen.

I explained the plots to no avail. He would shake his head, push himself to his feet, and head to the kitchen.

"Doesn't make any sense to me," he said, and pulled open his word puzzle book.

Thank you, God, that Dave has something to keep his mind busy, I often prayed.

It came as a relief to be able to turn down the blaring sound (necessary for Dave to hear the dialogue) to a more comfortable level for my sensitive ears. I watched the programs. He worked on his word puzzles. So our life settled down into a comfortable routine broken only by Dave's occasional health problems. We were barely existing, not really living, during those long years after we finally stopped losing family members to death.

CHAPTER 33

Doctor, Doctor, Doctor

One health problem we couldn't seem to conquer was Dave's weeping sores on his shin bones. In June of 2014, Dave had his annual visit to the heart doctor in Erie. After the usual pacemaker tests and ultra-sound of his heart, we waited for the doctor in what we thought would be the final exam room of the day. After his doctor consulted a nearby computer for Dave's test results, he smiled.

"Everything looks good, Mr. Bauer."

Then I pointed out those ugly sores on Dave's legs.

"We have tried everything, Doctor, but those sores keep coming back."

Doctor ordered a circulation test on the arteries in Dave's legs. Because we had such a long commute to Erie (180 miles round trip), the lab that conducted those tests made room for Dave that day. It seemed to take forever before the lab tech finished her probing needle and ultra-sound tests on Dave's sensitive legs. He grimaced several times, and finally protested.

"That hurts, you know."

She smiled brightly.

"That's a good thing, Mr. Bauer. It shows you still have feeling in your legs. If they were numb, we might have to operate today."

Just the word *operate* stunned Dave. Operate meant a hospital stay and he hated even thinking about that possibility. The pacemaker replacement, a fairly minor surgery performed last February, had been a nightmare for both of us. He shook his head.

"No operation!"

She patted his hand. "You won't have to stay overnight, and we do it right here in the doctor's suite."

He was still shaking his head when the doctor walked into the exam room. Somehow the doctor managed to talk Dave into having the minor surgery. It meant planning ahead. Dave would need blood work done, and come back to Erie another day for the procedure. We were both glad to leave St. Vincent's health complex and head home. On the way through Erie, we stopped at our favorite restaurant for supper. We both ate well, if silently. Dave didn't say much on the way home. I knew he hated the very thought of returning to Erie for yet another invasive procedure.

"Look at it this way, Dave. If it means your legs heal up, no more bloody socks and sheets, then why not? Doctor said it is no big deal."

Dave muttered to his lap.

"Every time I have to go to the hospital is a big deal to me."

The procedure was scheduled for the following Wednesday. On Monday of that week, he needed to have a fasting blood test at our local hospital. Usually, for fasting blood work, we would arise early and head for the laboratory as soon as it opened at 7 a.m. That way, the lack of breakfast wouldn't put him in trouble due to his diabetes. After the blood test, we went to a nearby Perkins to eat. Dave wasn't afraid of needles. He just hated to skip breakfast and head to the hospital for the test.

That Monday morning, I arose early and grabbed a quick snack so I wouldn't get shaky driving into town. Dave had slept in his recliner, which seemed to be happening more and more as he aged. I went over to his chair and kissed the top of his head.

"Time to get up, Dave. We need to hit the Lab early, remember?"

He stirred briefly then went back to sleep. I shook him several times, but he seemed glued to his chair that day. I planted my hands on my hips.

"Well, if you want to get good and hungry, sleep on, Bud."

Still no reaction. Just a turning away into sleep once again.

I drew a deep breath, praying for an avocado of patience.

"Guess I'll take the dog out for his walk. You better be ready to go when we get back."

Back home, I found Dave still glued to his chair.

Stubborn!

"Let me know when you are ready to go to town."

I turned to walk upstairs to my computer and play a game or two. No use fighting with a mule. He would get up sooner or later. Except he didn't. It was going on 10 a.m. and still Dave lingered in his chair. He barely protested as I took a finger prick to test his glucose level. A little low, but not dangerous. When I brought out the blood pressure cuff, he fought me off.

"Just leave me alone."

Something was just not right. Dave should be hungry by now. He never missed a meal. Now he refused to even stir out of his chair. Was it stubbornness? Fears about the thought of another surgery in two days? What?

"What is wrong with you?"

"Nothing. Leave me sleep!"

Now I was worried. Something might really be wrong. I tried a threat to get him moving.

"Dave, either you get up right now or I call 911."

Cursing and shaking his fists, he fought me off.

"Don't even think about calling the ambulance."

I called the ambulance. They arrived shortly, and the EMTs began assessing Dave's vital signs. He cursed them, swinging his fists as they took his vital signs.

"Mr. Bauer. You are sick. You have a fever of 102 degrees. You need to go to the hospital."

The fever surprised me.

"He wasn't warm when I kissed him this morning."

"What time was that?"

"Six-thirty."

"Well, since that time, his temperature has spiked to fever level. He needs medical attention, now."

I nodded, shocked. The men struggled to put Dave on a gurney. He swung his fists and kicked at them, cursing.

"You'll have to restrain him," I said faintly. "He has a terrible fear of hospitals."

Dave glared up at me with such hate in his eyes it felt like a blow from one of his clenched fists. I backed up. I had never seen such hate reflected in my beloved husband's eyes.

What is happening? Has his Alzheimer's disease reduced him to a man filled with unreasonable rage?

I bit my lips to keep from weeping as they carried Dave out to the waiting ambulance. It took the EMT's a long time to attend Dave in our driveway. They must have subdued him with something because at the Emergency Room, he lay comatose on the table. Above his head, machines tracked his blood pressure, heart rhythms, and pulse. I noticed his pulse rate was sinking below 50 and alerted the nurse.

"My husband's pacemaker is set at 70. It paces all the time. Now his reading is down to 50!"

She frowned. "How old is his pacemaker? Maybe the battery …?"

"Dave had a new pacemaker installed in February, four months ago. It is paced at 70, all the time."

She scrubbed his chest with the knuckles of one hand.

"Come on, Dave. Wake up now. Show a little life for me."

When the nurse mentioned a little life, my heart sank.

Is this it? Is he dying right before my eyes?

I stood up and leaned over my husband, ready to kiss him good-bye. Tears dripped on the sheet. Beside the bed, the monitor beeped out a regular rhythm. His pulse rate jumped to sixty, then, finally, to his normal paced rate of 70. Badly shaken, I sat down again.

A resident doctor pawed his way through the curtain surrounding Dave's bed. He read from a clipboard held in his hands.

"Mrs. Bauer?" I nodded. "Dave has sepsis, blood poisoning." He scratched his head and frowned. "Do you keep animals?"

"Just the family dog. Why?"

"Because there is some strain of animal material in this type of sepsis."

"Could it be because Dave allows the dog to lick his hands?"

The doctor scowled as he turned to the nurse.

"Give him an IV with a strong dose of antibiotic. It will take more than Cipro this time."

After hooking him up to an IV antibiotic drip, they admitted Dave to the hospital.

Whew! *Thank you, God, for saving my husband, yet again.*

I sat beside Dave as he gradually regained awareness. His anger seemed to have faded enough that he would squeeze my hand. His way of apologizing for that horrible expression of hate aimed my way as the ambulance crew took him out of our living room. We sat quietly, rarely speaking, as twilight faded, replaced by evening darkness. I stayed with Dave until after he ate his supper, propped up in the hospital bed. He picked at the hospital food, frowning as he ate.

"Tastes awful," he said, but he ate everything on the tray and looked for more. He wanted me to stay overnight, but I reminded him that the dog needed his supper and his nightly walk. Reluctantly, he let go of my hand and sank back against the pillows.

"You coming back tomorrow?" he asked.

His eyes were frightened. Did he really believe I would abandon him at this late date, after sixty plus years of married life? I patted his hand and forced an exhausted smile.

"Of course. Where else would I go?"

That night I slept alone in our house, the house we built together so many years ago. My heart was heavy with the thought of the future. How many health problems could Dave survive before God took him home to heaven?

And what will I do if Dave dies and leaves me all alone?

It was not a good night's sleep, that night or for many nights after.

CHAPTER 34

The Bed Bath Fiasco

Next morning I gathered up a bundle of requested items to take with me to the hospital. As I dragged my load of medicine and equipment past the nurses' station, I stopped and leaned over the high counter.

"So, did Dave behave himself last night?"

The nurses rolled their eyes. No one answered.

"OK, I get it," I said and continued down the hallway to his room.

Even before I reached his room, I heard him bellowing. I heaved a long sigh and braced myself for whatever chaotic scene waited for me in Dave's room. My husband sat on a bedside commode, nude except for a towel across his lap. An aide struggled with a washcloth, trying to wash Dave's back. She was pretty good at dodging his fists and even managed to laugh at his outraged bellowing.

"Now, Mr. Bauer. I'm only trying to clean you up a little. A little soap and water won't kill you."

I set down my bags, purse, water bottle, and lunch tote. Leaning my cane against the wall, I reached for the wash cloth. She gave it up willingly.

"Let me try. He really hates being wet. Especially a drippy wash cloth."

"And it's a *cold* wash cloth," Dave yelled.

I dipped the cloth in the nice warm water and wrung it out thoroughly.

"See Hon, it's not so bad. Let me wash your back now."

He leaned forward with a long sigh.

"I thought you would never get here. They're trying to freeze me to death."

He scowled at the aide.

I turned to offer an apology to the woman as I rubbed Dave's back with the warm cloth. As I straightened up, my elbow landed in the pan of water on the bedside table. Oops! A cascade of soapy water landed all over Dave, me, and the aide. Dave erupted, arms waving, eyes bulging, mouth screaming.

"You trying to drown me?"

The aide snickered. I laughed so hard I had to sit on the edge of the bed to keep from falling into Dave's outraged arms.

"I'm sorry! I'm sorry!"

I kept apologizing as I frantically blotted water off Dave with a nearby towel. But I couldn't stop laughing. The aide managed to soak up most of the spilled water off her patient and the floor. This is the scene the resident doctor saw as she swept into the room, followed by her entourage of interns. These young doctors absorbed her every word, nodding at each decision as if she were the Queen of the Universe.

"Well, Mr. Bauer," she pronounced regally.

She stared at the chaotic scene before her. Dave, shivering on a bedside commode, the spilled water around him, and the merriment of both the aide and me.

"Looks like you will be going home today."

Finally, finally, something made Dave smile.

As the doctor swept out of the room, I hurried after her.

"What did Dave's CT scan show?" I asked, worried about another stroke.

Her Highness didn't even turn around to grace me with a glance.

"Looked normal. He can go home today. The floor nurse will give you the paperwork."

I almost curtsied. Better than screaming at her for her obvious lack of interest in my beloved husband's health, ya think? At least I could take Dave home, which made him very happy, indeed. Later at home, I canceled his artery surgery scheduled for the next day in Erie.

Dave never did have to endure another trip to Erie for surgery. Because later that week, consulting with various doctors, we put Dave in Hospice care.

CHAPTER 35

Hospice: Miracle Workers

Once Dave had been accepted into Hospice care our lives improved greatly. Nurses came several times a week to dress his bleeding legs. Within weeks his legs were clean, healed by the special bandages and salves provided by Hospice. His medications were delivered to the house, no charge, paid for by the program. A social worker came, *for me!* To help me manage Dave's moods and weird silences. We signed up for Meals on Wheels and that eliminated a big job for me. Now I could devote more time and attention to Dave's needs rather than trying to dream up a meal that my husband would actually eat. A housekeeper came once a week to vacuum for me, a true back saver. As I aged, my back grew weaker. Now I could sit back, keep Dave company elsewhere, while the vacuum whined in the main part of the house. Sometimes, he came upstairs so I could show him funny videos on Facebook, and let him see the pictures posted by our big extended family.

At first he seemed happy to watch the computer monitor, but later he complained it took too much out of him to climb the stairs to my computer room. He would take the dog and sulk in our bedroom as the very nice lady vacuumed the rest of the house. I shrugged off his moods. If I let it get to me, all those dark glances and muttering complaints, I would grow even more depressed. As it was, it often took all of my avocado seed of patience to even make it through the day without yelling at him. He seldom took any dog walks, so that chore fell to me too. I welcomed the time out of the house as my private prayer time. I called the dog walk, my rosary walk, because that has always been my go-to prayer every day. Still is.

Thank you, Mary, holy Mother of Jesus, for giving your beautiful prayer, the rosary, to the people of earth.

Summer warmth finally stirred Dave to action. He began to ride the mower again, an activity that soothed him, made him feel useful again. He took his time cutting the lawn and the field paths I used for my daily dog walks. His face looked relaxed, his mood mellow, as round and round he drove. *Doing something useful, something manly,* a throwback to his farm-boy youth when he used to plow acres of his father's land using a two horse team and a walk-behind plow.

The visiting nurse did not approve of Dave riding his machine.

"Aren't you afraid he might hurt himself, Mrs. Bauer?"

I smiled. "It makes him happy. Besides, even if he falls asleep and runs into a tree, he wouldn't get hurt. He drives so slowly, even if he fell off, he wouldn't hurt himself. The seat on his tractor is a safety seat. It shuts off as soon as his weight is lifted off."

Nurse was not happy, but I would not forbid my husband from doing the one thing that brought him joy those long troubled days.

One day I did have second thoughts about Dave's love affair with his riding mower. It happened on a late afternoon. It was almost time to start supper when I glanced out the back door. Dave was sitting hunched over the steering wheel of the lawn tractor, fast asleep. I went out to wake him up.

"Almost supper time, Dave. Time to put your toy away and come inside."

He lifted his head and glared at me.

"I'm fine right here."

"Dave! It's hot out here. You will get a heat stroke sitting in the sun like this. Park the mower and come inside."

"No! And you can't make me."

Oh dear, now my avocado seed of patience zipped out of my hands and flew the coop. Trouble ahead. I folded my arms and matched him glare for glare. He reminded me of a stubborn toddler, hanging onto a favorite toy, refusing to listen to reason. Reminded me of Baby Boy, clinging to his Brumm-brumm in the store until I bought it for him. Now I faced a similar standoff between me and my stubborn husband. I marched into the house, grabbed the keys to his 4-wheeler, slipped them and the keys to the car in my pocket, and stomped back down the steps outside.

"Last chance. Are you coming inside? Now!"

Down went his head over the steering wheel of the lawn mower.

Without another word, I reached across him and snagged the keys to the mower. Moments later, I jumped into the car and roared out of the garage. I did take a tour around the back of the house in order to beep the horn. When Dave glanced up, surprised, I waved.

"Bye-bye."

Scenes like this are called caregiver burnout. Without any of our adult children or grandchildren living nearby, I had no one to call on when I needed a break from troubling situations, familiar to anyone dealing with an Alzheimer's patient. I made sure Dave had no means of transportation before I left, taking our only car, and the keys to the lawn mower and the ATV.

I drove out the lane, wondering just where to go to cool off. My husband could be so maddening! I don't like fighting or loud scenes with shouted words hurled at loved ones. Cruel words might never be forgotten, nor forgiven. Far better to just disappear for a while, I believe. Aimlessly I drove down the lane and turned right.

I kept driving, my mind numb, heart fearful of what problems lay ahead for Dave and me. If I couldn't even get him to come into the house at supper time, how would I take care of him later, when his mind slipped away completely? Finally, I ended up at my friend Kay's house. Thankfully she was at home and welcomed me inside. One look at my thunderous expression and she guessed we had problems at home, but she asked no questions. I spent a couple of hours with Kay and another friend who dropped by later. We talked about various happy things, not problems. The time passed quickly and pleasantly. Kay's husband stayed in the kitchen as he prepared their evening meal. When he poked his head around the corner and invited me to stay for supper, I realized it was time to leave.

I hugged everyone available, thanked them, and left to go home.

The mower still sat in the yard but the seat was empty. Inside, I found Dave sulking in his recliner, pretending to be asleep. I fixed a peanut butter and jam sandwich for my supper, then went upstairs to play computer games until bedtime. The sounds of cupboard doors slamming in the kitchen alerted me that Dave had taken the hint and made himself something to eat.

Did he really think I would cook for him after the way he acted?

Apparently so, but he had another think coming, as his Mum used to say.

After that tough lesson, no more mulish behavior from Mr. Stubborn Butt.

CHAPTER 36

Autumn, 2014

Our daily schedule was governed by the nursing schedule of Hospice. It kept Dave centered, happy to be fussed over by the nice people from the Visiting Nurses Association (VNA). He continued to do outside work, mowing, raking leaves, burning the blow-down limbs from our trees. Northwestern Pennsylvania hosts a lot of high wind storms during all seasons of the year. Dave kept the fallen limbs and debris picked up and piled in our fire ring at the top of our property. Usually, the day after we had a soaking rainstorm, Dave would deem it a perfect time to burn the forest trash. He loved to sit in a lawn chair and watch the waste wood burn. Might have reminded him of our camping days, long ago, when our family was young.

"Anybody got any marshmallows?"

At lunch time, he returned to the house, smelling of wood smoke, a contented expression on his tired face. Afternoons were for napping.

As the season slid into late autumn, he began to harvest the apples from our three trees. One tree, an Ida Red, provided plenty of winter apples that year. These beautiful apples, tinted a deep red, grew large and luscious as they hung from the very top of the tree. No matter how hard Dave shook the tree trunk or its lower branches, the apples on the highest limbs refused to fall. I went out one afternoon to help him. We had several extension poles in the garage. They were aluminum, but still heavy. It took both of us to hang onto the lowest part of the pole, lift up and rattle the upper limbs. Apples rained down upon us. Dave lost his grip on the pole. Without his help, I couldn't hold on and the pole crashed to the ground. I ducked and laughed as an apple thumped me on top of my head. Rubbing my head, I glanced around.

Dave lay on his back among the rhubarb stalks, arms outstretched as apples pelted him from above. He kept grinning and dodging our fruitful bounty.

"Pretty good crop this year, right Hon?" he said, smiling.

The downed apples filled a five gallon bucket and more. Months later, after his death, I made apple pie from the last of those autumn beauties. As I peeled and sliced the apples, my mind strayed back to a golden autumn day. Dave lying in the grass beneath our apple trees, looking up and laughing as the fruit rained down on him.

Thank you God, for golden memories. And for Ida Red apples made into delicious pies.

CHAPTER 37

Dave's Project

Sometime during that autumn, Dave decided to build a new cover for our mulch pile. The old mulchie, as we called it, had been fashioned from small logs arranged in a square, topped by a strong screened cover. The screen kept out animals including Smokey. We used it to recycle our kitchen peelings and coffee grounds. Whenever Dave set out to build something new, he tended to fret about it for long periods of indecision. Should he use other logs for the base? Maybe he needed to buy some new lumber, 2x4's or perhaps 2x6's to form a sturdy framework? What about the top? A screen or what?

I would find him in the garage pacing around, pausing to stare at his scrap lumber pile, tapping his foot, as he struggled to make a decision and actually begin making something to suit the occasion. Finally I made a suggestion. He was so touchy these days. I hated to upset him and bring on another tantrum.

"Hey Dave? How about using that old screen door you built years ago."

This had been our first screen door before we replaced it with an aluminum storm door. I pointed toward the rafters of the garage where the wooden door had been stored across the open beams. He looked up. A thoughtful expression shadowed his face. Encouraged, I continued.

"You could build a support frame around that old door out of some of your scrap lumber. A lot less work than starting from scratch, ya think?"

Dave nodded and gave me a grateful glance. We worked together to bring the screen door down. He climbed a stepladder. I held the ladder steady so he wouldn't take another dive onto the garage floor. He slid the door across the rafters until it tipped toward me. I reached up and grabbed the edge and held it until he descended the ladder.

At last! He had a plan and I had helped him without stirring up his anger.

He grabbed a tape measure off the workbench and began jotting down numbers. Funny thing about old farm boys. They don't use paper to record their measurements. They grab up scraps of wood instead. It was a common thing to see Dave carrying around a small piece of lumber with numbers scrawled across every surface.

Whatever works, I thought, happy he had the will and the ideas to begin working on his project. I retreated into the house, grateful I had been able to get him started.

Thanks God, for helping me with Dave.

It was a prayer I uttered silently each day as I leaned on God to help me with the difficult "handling" of my troubled husband.

Later that afternoon, I listened to the muted sound of the table saw Dave kept in his garage workshop. It ran briefly, then shut off. This happened several times without incident. I tried not to worry about Dave using such a powerful tool. He had always been super careful with the big saw. Without fail, he used a guide and a "pusher'" a scrap of wood that helped push the wood through the saw blade. So when Dave came into the house and headed for the kitchen sink, I assumed he was washing up for supper. Then I noticed the blood on his sleeve.

"What happened?"

I rushed to his side, almost afraid to look at his hands or arms. He shrugged and turned away, trying to prevent me from seeing his left index finger.

"Oh, nothing to get excited about," he said. "Saw nicked my finger, that's all."

I wriggled around him until I could see his hand as he held his finger under the running water. His index finger had several scratch-like wounds around it.

"Doesn't look too bad, Dave."

He grinned.

"Yeah, just a nick here and there. Guess I forgot to use the pusher."

I bandaged him up without comment. I knew if I pitched a fit about his "forgetting" the most basic safety rules about operating a table saw, he would just hop up on his high horse and get all blustery about the accident. *And go out and do it all again, just to show me he was boss!*

The next day, the Hospice nurse was not so understanding when she examined Dave's wound. She frowned at both of us.

"Dave! You have no idea how badly this might have turned out. You could have lost this finger or even your whole hand." She shook her finger under Dave's nose. "I don't want you working in the garage again! You hear me?"

She glared at me, then.

"What were you thinking allowing Dave around power tools?"

I shrugged and spread my hands. My husband outweighed me by sixty pounds. How was I supposed to control him? I didn't own a Taser.

"You do realize that Dave won't listen to me? What am I supposed to do, shoot him?"

It was an empty threat, as I am sure the nurse knew. A brief warning to other families with firearms. When caring for a loved one with Alzheimer's, make sure all your guns are locked up with the keys safely hidden. In our case, Dave's arsenal of hunting weapons were all unloaded, the shells safely stashed away in a hidden container. The key to the gun cabinet lived in my pocket. I took these precautions months before, when Dave first showed signs of uncontrolled anger.

The nurse gave me a long stare, heaved a sigh and wrote something in her notebook. Before she left that day, the nurse repeated her order to Dave.

"No more working in the garage!"

Surprisingly, he obeyed her. He no longer worked in the garage. But he did not give up on his project, either. He simply dragged the whole assembly out onto the grass beside the garage and worked from there.

That evening, I relaxed in my recliner and watched a program on TV. I heard Dave's power drill as he assembled framework for the new mulchie cover. Later, he came into the kitchen and went to the sink. I heard water running, then Dave called me.

"Can you come and see what's in my ear?"

As I walked toward the kitchen, I assumed a fly or other bug had flown into Dave's ear. When I rounded the corner and saw all the blood, my heart gave a big leap of fear. I had not heard the big saw running. What happened?

Dave's right ear dripped a red river down his face. His hands, arms and shirt were drenched with bright red blood. Even after raising ten children and nursing all their various bloody injuries, the sight of my husband's blood running into the kitchen sink made me feel faint.

"Dave? What on earth?"

He looked pretty pale, too. The sight of all that blood, *his blood*, made his voice quaver.

"I tripped and fell into the screen door. Guess the screen sliced me up pretty bad."

His earlobe had been sliced open from the edge of his ear to the tip of the lobe. I grabbed a big towel, pressed it onto his ear, and helped him sit on a kitchen chair. Grabbing my cell phone, I speed dialed the nurse. She was on her way home, but she turned around and came back to assess Dave's newest injury. I had hoped she had some skin glue in her bag to put Dave's ear back together. No such luck. He needed to go to the Emergency Room. *A hospital visit.* I braced myself for a king sized tantrum from my volatile husband. But Dave surprised me. Meekly he listened as the nurse explained she could not help him at home. He really needed to go to the ER for professional help.

"You won't have to stay overnight, I promise."

He nodded, his face pale with fear.

Bless that knowledgeable nurse. She phoned ahead to the hospital, explained Dave's phobia about hospitals, and even offered to drive him there. Fortunately, he agreed to ride with me. Once at the Emergency department, Dave was whisked into a private room. No curtains around his bed. No noisy hustle and bustle of a busy ER facility. Just a wonderfully quiet room where he and I could sit side by side as he waited to be stitched up. Two doctors worked over him quickly and quietly. We had to stay for a while to make sure Dave didn't go into shock. It was close to midnight before they released him. He hadn't said two words since I wheeled him into the hospital. Now he sat beside me in the car.

"How do you feel?" I asked, sticking the key in the ignition.

"Hungry."

Walmart was just a short distance away. I parked in Handicapped, ran into the store, grabbed up the nearest box of donuts, hit the register, and raced out again.

"Here you go, Hon. Help yourself."

"I'll wait till we get home. Hate to make a mess in the car."

His voice was gruff, but not angry. I think he was mighty relieved to be going home instead of being cooped up in a hospital again. We had a late night snack of donuts before staggering off to bed. Dave, of course, shared his donuts with Smokey.

Ten days later, a Hospice doctor came out to the house and plucked out the ten stitches within Dave's ear.

And yes, he did finish the mulchie cover. It stands in the woods beside the garage. Every time I use it, I remember Dave and his last building project.

CHAPTER 38

The Fading Days

Thanksgiving went by in a blur. We had a houseful of people including Rose's family, and Dave's brother, John, plus their sister Betty. Flo prepared the dinner, chicken and rice, plus cranberry sauce. I always made coleslaw for holidays. Flo was an avid fan of my slaw, so I made it for him in thanksgiving for all his culinary skills in my kitchen. Dave's health problems kept me so busy, I had little time or energy to prepare a big holiday meal. Weeks before Thanksgiving, I told Rose, "I've cooked my last turkey."

Thank you God, for generous loving family members.

Dave ate well as we all did. He even enjoyed two pieces of pie. After dinner, as the rest of us cleared up the table and put away leftovers, Dave dozed off in his recliner. He slept all evening, not ever stirring to give hugs good-bye as our families left for home. Rose's face looked drawn as she gazed at her sleeping father. Unhappy fears glistened in her eyes. She hugged me extra hard.

"Let me know if you need help, Mom," she whispered. "I can take time off from work ..."

I nodded, but I knew she had just started a new job, a good job. I vowed I would not jeopardize her new position unless something drastic happened with her father.

Toward the end of November, at the request of the visiting nurse, I began keeping a journal of Dave's worsening symptoms as the real Dave faded and an angry stranger took his place.

November 29:

Seemed sluggish this morning. He forgot to take his pills at lunch time. He woke up from a nap very confused.

"What's going on?" he said, staring around as if he did not recognize our living room.

I struggled to remain calm. To try to reason with him when he showed confusion, only made him angry. Calm was what I strived for each day, each moment of our long journey together toward the inevitable end of Dave's mental and physical struggles here on earth.

"Almost supper time," I said. "Time for you to take the dog out for a walk, before it gets dark."

"What? Where do we go?"

Reluctantly he donned his winter coat. It took him a long while to get the zipper up and find his heavy gloves. The dog danced around his feet, waiting impatiently for their daily walk. They stepped out the door together and walked down the ramp. Dave kept staring around at the snow-covered yard. The bird feeder caught his attention for long moments. Smokey barked for attention, dancing on the walk path, trying to entice Dave into their usual routine. Finally, Dave took a few steps toward the path. I left the window and prepared supper. Time passed.

They should be back by now. I looked out the window. No sign of man nor beast. Sighing, I pulled on my boots, coat and gloves, and headed out the back door. Dave stood at the top of our property hidden from view by several trees. He stood there like a stranger in purgatory, staring around, a frightened expression on his face. Smokey sat at his feet, staring up at his master's face. I took Dave's arm.

"Supper is ready," I said, urging him toward the house.

He came without a struggle, happy, I think, for my guidance. *How frightening it must be for him*, I thought. He didn't even remember how to come home anymore. He did eat well, a now rare occasion, and fell asleep at the table, his nose in a word puzzle magazine.

Two hours later, I roused him.

"Come on, Dear. You need a bath. It's been a while since you cleaned up. I will help you."

One of the first casualties in a dementia patient's everyday life is personal hygiene. He was combative as I helped him undress for a chair bath. He flung his clothing onto the floor and cussed me out at every move. The sponge bath was a nightmare of complaints, moans and groans.

"It's too cold for a bath. You're trying to drown me again!"

I dodged his fists and kept undressing him. A large bruise decorated his back. His shoulder sported a long scratch. The wounds were old enough that they were half healed.

"What happened, Dave?"

He shrugged and looked at his feet. I applied antibiotic ointment. He insisted on seeing the tube before he would allow me to doctor up his scrapes.

"What? You think I'm out to get you with a tube of salve?"

His shrug made me mad. I clammed up. Dave protested as I tried to re-dress him in a clean white tee shirt. He did not recognize it.

"That's not my shirt. I wear colored shirts, not this one. What did you do with my real shirts?"

"Tomorrow is Sunday. You always wear white undershirts on Sunday to go with your dress shirts."

"Not going to church anymore!"

"Whatever. You still have to wear this shirt. All the colored shirts are in the hamper."

After a long exhausting struggle he was dressed and headed for his recliner. He slept all night in his chair, his tongue sticking out one corner of his mouth. Sleeping in his recliner seemed to help him rest better than lying beside me in our bed. I covered him with a second blanket before I turned out most of the lights. Night-lights kept the darkness at bay in case Dave needed to use the bathroom.

Another day over without a screaming argument. Thank you, God, for that avocado of patience. Really need that these days.

The next day, Sunday, I tried to wake him up for breakfast. He refused to open his eyes or acknowledge me at all. Maybe he held a grudge about having to wear the wrong color tee shirt? His tongue, sticking out the corner of his mouth, looked dry, caked with thick drool. When he didn't respond to my shaking him, I brought out the diabetes test kit. His glucose measured 74, a bit low. Anything between 80 to 120 was considered normal. I gave him two glucose sugar tabs, sliding them past his tongue. Even if he was sound asleep, the tabs would dissolve and help raise his sugar number. Fifteen minutes later, when Smokey and I returned from the morning dog walk, Dave was up and in the bathroom. He fell asleep in there, too. I woke him for breakfast. He sat at the table eating his eggs and homemade bread as I kissed him goodbye and headed off to church.

God? How much of Dave's behavior is due to his illness, and how much of it is just his way of yanking my chain? Desperately need that avocado of patience, please God?

CHAPTER 39

Too Brief Visits from the Real Dave

Later that same Sunday, I woke Dave for supper.

"Could you set the table for me, Hon?"

He stood in the kitchen and stared at the table, unable to grasp the concept of taking two plates and two sets of silverware out of the nearby cupboard and laying them on the table. He glanced up at me, confused and embarrassed.

"Time to pray?" he asked.

I nodded, as I set the table around his hulking figure.

"Yep, supper time."

Must still be half asleep, I thought. In those days, I often rationalized my husband's odd behavior. It seemed easier than facing the reality of his accelerating mental decline.

After he ate, and he did eat well that Sunday evening, he fell asleep at table. He slept for three hours, often leaning forward until his nose touched his knees. I tried to wake him so he might move to his recliner, but he ignored my pleas and slept on. Yet, at 8 p.m., he roused himself, climbed to his feet, stood a moment to regain his balance, then moved to the freezer to bring out his ice cream. Dave, just like our son Russ, loved his sweet treats. He dished up a large portion, ate half of it, and gave the rest to the dog. After another long nap in the bathroom, he climbed into bed beside me and slept well all night.

The next morning, we both rejoiced in the real Dave's return. He even made a joke before sitting down to a hearty breakfast of eggs and homemade bread. All day, the real Dave reigned in our suddenly normal home. After supper, things changed. His eyes reflected confusion as he puzzled over his word-finder book.

"This doesn't make sense," he said, tapping the pages.

"Maybe you need some fresh air? Might wake you up?"

He watched as I gathered up paper garbage to burn. Suddenly, he stood up.

"Let me do that! I can burn the garbage."

He sat down in the back hall/laundry room and pulled on his boots. It didn't seem to take him as long to zipper up his thick winter coat. Some days, this was a heartbreaking ritual to watch as he struggled with numb fingers to fit the sides of the long zipper together. Often I had to help him, but not tonight. That evening, he seemed more competent as he dressed himself for outdoors.

He pulled on his gloves and patted his pocket where his lighter lived. Grabbing the plastic bag of paper waste, he headed out the door toward the burn barrel. Smokey followed him, happy to be hanging out with his favorite master. I sat at the kitchen window and watched as Dave used the lighter. The bag began to burn. He stepped away, leaning on the long poker he kept nearby. Occasionally, he would step closer to the barrel and poke at the garbage as it burned. I watched for several minutes, then took a quick bathroom break.

When I returned to the window, Dave had disappeared! *What happened?*

Alarmed, I hurried toward the back door just as Dave stomped up the ramp. He lurched into the house in a rage. He had fallen asleep while standing beside the barrel. Thank God he had fallen to the side instead of into the fire. His right hip and legs were muddy. He gestured toward his messy pants and glared at me. Somehow this was *all my fault*. I didn't argue with him about this. Blaming me whenever something bad happened had been his pattern for years. Usually, I reminded him that I was not responsible for his mistakes. But that night the blame game did not bother me. It almost seemed normal. The upside of his latest accident meant I had an opportunity to wash him up and change his clothing. Exhausted by his misadventure, he slept through the night, in our bed. Yay! The next day, real Dave returned. He even swept the kitchen floor, and offered to dry the dishes for me.

As the month of December continued, Dave's confused days were more frequent than his real Dave days. I noticed he often needed reminders to take his medications. Previously, Dave had always been in charge of his pill routine. Now he had trouble recognizing the medication. He would stare at the labels, frowning, and put them down again. Only to pick up another bottle and repeat the routine. Stare at the label, shake the pills inside, then put the bottle down again. Finally, I brought out the pill container that Russ used during his final illness. It had slots for morning, noon, evening and night medication. I sat beside Dave, checking the medication list we kept on the refrigerator and sorting out the various pills into the proper slots. He accepted this routine at first. Later he refused to take a pill if he didn't recognize the shape or color.

He became increasingly suspicious of me and my motives. This began in October when the local Sheriff came out to the house to put a GPS bracelet on Dave's wrist. I had explained its purpose to him numerous times. I worried whenever he took the dog out for a walk. Tall corn fields surrounded our property. Dave had only to stumble and fall into one of those endless fields of unharvested corn and I would never find him again. An elderly man had died this way a few months back. I did not want to become a corn widow.

Reluctantly, Dave allowed the Sheriff to put the bracelet on his wrist. He was not enthused about it but he went along with it so, "You won't be so worried all the time."

I hugged him and told him many times that day how much I appreciated his wearing the bracelet. *Thank you, God, that Dave still loves me despite his confusion.*

But as December wore on, the bracelet really bugged him. He often plucked at it, a deep scowl on his face. I wondered just how long he would endure it before he would tear it off in a rage and stomp it into the snow and mud outside.

One evening, we attended Mass at our church. It was a holy day, and also daughter Rose's birthday. I had called to wish her a happy birthday before we left for church. Good thing, because Dave would have been so embarrassed if I had called her after Mass and told her what happened that night.

Mass began at 7 p.m. Because it was December 8th, it was winter dark when we walked out of church. Our new pastor, Father Christopher, always stood outside in the parking lot to shake hands with the people coming out of church. Four steps lead from the church's main floor to the parking lot. Dave, carefully using his cane, missed a step and fell forward. Father opened his arms and Dave stumbled right into them. Our pastor laughed at the unexpected hug. Dave was mortified. He hated the idea that he had made a spectacle of himself by falling into the priest. He apologized over and over. Neither man was injured, so no harm, no foul, I thought. But Dave felt humiliated. For the next several weeks, he refused to go to Mass at all.

Lord, forgive me for not being more sympathetic
to my husband's feelings.

CHAPTER 40

No More Real Dave

Friday, December 12th: Another sleepy day for Dave. He seemed to spend a lot of time unconscious in his recliner or at the kitchen table sleeping with his face down on the table. Midmorning, as awoke to go to the bathroom, I handed him a dirty kitchen towel.

"Could you toss this in the washer for me, Hon?"

He stopped mid-stride in the laundry room. He stared at the towel in his hand. His eyes were vague, confused, as he lifted the towel to his face and examined it carefully. He turned to me, seemingly frozen in time.

"What?"

Impatient, I grabbed up the towel and tossed it in the washer. He stared at me, bewildered.

"Never mind," I said, and gently nudged him toward the bathroom. "Don't you need to go now?"

He shrugged and spread his hands, a gesture I used to hate because he had always used it to end any argument between us. It meant, *I know that I am right in this matter, but I bow to you, my nagging wife, to keep the peace.* Now this familiar gesture made my heart hurt.

God, Dave has lost so much of himself. Please bless him today.

After his bathroom visit, he moved to the living room recliner and slept so soundly, even the high whining sound of the vacuum cleaner did not waken him. Later, after the noise stopped, Dave woke up and moved to our bedroom. When I checked later, I found him lying down on the bed. This was a most rare action on his part. He never used the bed for naps during the day. He stayed there, fully dressed, shoes and all, until the visiting nurse arrived. Even then, he didn't get up, but allowed her to check his vitals as he dozed off and on. The nurse glanced at me, trying to gauge my reaction to this rare event. She motioned me into another room.

"Is it time to order a hospital bed for the living room?" she said.

I shook my head although I really didn't have a clue what to do.

"Maybe later, if he decides to sleep on a bed from now on. Right now, he sleeps better sitting up in his recliner, or at the table." I sighed. "Or in the bathroom."

She typed something on her laptop computer.

"Has he taken any new falls?"

I thought of all the times Dave had fallen lately. I would be in bed for the night, almost asleep, when the loud thump and rattle of a body hitting the floor would alert me. Leaping out of bed, heart in my throat, I feared checking on Dave's safety. Those loud, house-rattling sounds of a body hitting the floor always made me imagine the worst.

Is this it? Did Dave die just now?

Reluctantly, I would open the bathroom door, only to find him on hands and knees, half-asleep, struggling to climb to his feet again.

"Guess I fell asleep," he said, sheepishly, every time this happened.

The nurse shook her head.

"Maybe he needs something to help him sleep soundly, *after* he gets settled for the night."

She talked to the hospice doctor and he approved a liquid sedative. I gave it to Dave once. He made a face at the bitter taste. But the medication did not help. In fact, it seemed to keep him wired, fully awake and more prone to falling than before.

December 13th: Dave and I embarked on a household project. The kitchen chairs needed new covers. The seat covers were made of upholstery material. They were too soiled now to be scrubbed clean. Time to replace them with fresh new covers. We had worked together on this type of project several times before.

Dave seemed to remember how to disassemble the seats by unscrewing several long screws underneath. He used a portable drill. I used a screwdriver. Somehow I managed to remove more screws than Dave did. It saddened me to see how much my husband had forgotten. He used to be Mr. Fix-it, ready for any challenging project. Now he struggled to handle his power drill. Yet together, we managed to re-cover one chair before Dave had a mental meltdown.

"Where is that other chair?" he said, counting and re-counting the remaining three chairs.

Thinking his glucose might be dropping, I handed him two mini candy bars. He sat down, munching thoughtfully, staring at nothing.

What goes on behind those dreamy eyes? I wondered. *God, please help him.*

As he rested, I lifted up the second chair, put it upside down on the edge of the table, and began removing screws. He stood up long enough to hold the new material in place as I finished replacing the screws.

"Two chairs done," I said. "Enough for today. We can do the rest tomorrow."

That evening he slept in his recliner until bedtime, then stayed up past midnight to work on his word-finder puzzles. I felt him crawl into bed in the middle of the night. I rolled toward him and curled around his frigid body. He seemed so cold these days, despite the super warmth of our house. Dave kept upping the thermostat until it read eighty degrees. Still he shivered day and night. My body has always been a super-heat conductor. It did its job and warmed Dave up until he stopped shivering and fell into a deep sleep.

Thank you, God, for the comfort of my husband beside me in our bed.

Sunday, December 15th: Dave did not want to get up that morning. I tried to rouse him for breakfast, but he refused to budge. His sleepy eyes reflected deep confusion.

"I lost my key!" he blurted. "I told Mum about it, but I can't find my key!"

Mum would be his mother, dead now for 40-plus years. When I reminded him that Mum died in 1970, he changed his story.

"I meant your mother. I told her about my key."

I sat on the edge of the bed and stroked his arm.

"Dave, my mother died in 1990. Remember we took care of her when she died of cancer?"

He did not appreciate me correcting him. Becoming agitated, he yelled.

"I mean my wife!"

"Your wife?" I had to laugh.

This made him even more angry.

"Yes, my wife! I told my wife!"

Sudden tears stung my eyes. I got up and left the bedroom.

His wife? Then what am I, chopped liver?

Fetching his glucose tester I checked his blood count. Seventy-four. Time for two glucose tabs. I felt torn about leaving him to go to church. By the time I put on my coat, he had fallen into a deep sleep. I risked leaving him alone to go to Mass. Halfway through Mass, I felt an unbearable nudge to *go home, now!* False alarm. Dave was still asleep, breathing normally and snoring. His blood pressure was a bit high, better than it bottoming out. He finally got up at ten and ate a normal breakfast. That evening he worked himself into a rage about the GPS bracelet on his wrist. He threatened to cut it off. We exchanged angry words, shouting at each other. I felt helpless, burned out. I wanted to walk out the door and never come back. But of course, a good wife, even when her husband doesn't recognize her, sticks it out through thick and thin.

Caregiver burnout. Please help me, O God.
I feel my avocado seed of much-needed patience
slipping away. Sustain me O God of heaven and earth.

CHAPTER 41

Miracle of the Sacraments

Saturday, December 20. After a slow start, Dave spent most of the day in his recliner, sound asleep. I called him twice for supper, then shouted my now familiar threat.

"Supper is on the table, and I don't deliver!"

Good news for today: Dave agreed to go to Marienville this evening for Mass so we both could go to Confession before the services began. I went into the "black box" first, confessed my sins, then asked our pastor to pray for me, since I had so much trouble being patient with Dave. I walked out that door, reassured that God had listened to my prayers and forgave me.

Dave's turn. He seemed reluctant, confused, as a church friend gently guided him through the confessional door. As the door closed, I prayed for Dave, realizing he might now be past the point where familiar rituals, such as the Sacraments of Penance, and Communion, registered in his cloudy mind. But Dave came out smiling, walking slowly toward me, his cane keeping him steady. He entered the pew and knelt down for a few minutes. When he relaxed into a sitting position, he leaned toward me to whisper.

"I told Father I was sorry for trying to knock him down that time outside church."

I smiled, knowing full well that no sin had been committed in my husband's accidental stumble into Father's arms. Dave smiled too. He seemed so relaxed and relieved now. I breathed a long sigh of relief and said a quick prayer of thanksgiving. During Communion time, he gladly stood up and followed me toward the front of the church to receive the Body of Christ.

Receiving those two Sacraments seemed to help Dave's mood all that evening. Absent was the familiar scowl he often wore now as his mind played tricks on his good intentions. But the next day, confusion reigned again. He thought it was Monday and wondered aloud what happened to the daily paper, which had no Sunday delivery.

"Those darn kids!" he said, striking one fist into the other. "Stealing our paper! You better do something about this."

Wearily, I nodded. What use arguing with him? I did wonder which darn kids he meant.

"The paper will come tomorrow," I told him.

He stared at me for long moments. "You sure?"

I nodded. He sat back on his recliner and fell into a deep sleep. When I woke him up for lunch, he thought it was supper time. But, he did volunteer to take the dog out for a walk later, before supper. This was noteworthy. More and more dog walking became my job as the weather turned nasty. Dave hated the cold. Best of all that evening, he and the dog returned ravenous, and both enjoyed their supper. Dave even dried the dishes for me.

Thank you, God, for sending my real Dave back for a visit.

Wednesday, December 23. Visiting nurse came, checked Dave's vitals, and treated his legs with ointment and special compression bandages called tuba-grips. After she left, Dave went down cellar as I prepared lunch. He intended to wash off a soiled throw rug using the spray hose attached to the sink in my basement kitchen area. As I put his pills on the table, strange sounds echoed up the stairway.

I heard the clang of the 3-step ladder as it hit the concrete floor. Then the rattle of the bag of crushed aluminum cans, kept on the pool table. Worst of all was the sound of a loud thump as his body rolled off the pool table and onto the cement floor. His groan sent me hurtling down the steps. I found him on his back holding his head. His eyes were cloudy with confusion. He was disoriented as he accepted my help to climb to his feet. Weaving, he staggered up the cellar stairway and into the kitchen. His body shook as he collapsed into the kitchen chair. His speech rambled as he stared around, looking for "C.O." He waved away my offer of lunch items.

"C.O. I want C.O."

He stared down at his empty plate, waiting for the elusive item stuck in his confused mind.

I brought out every food item I could thing of beginning with the letter C: cheese, coffee, candy, cupcake?

He shook his head over and over again.

"C.O. I want C.O.!"

Finally, disgusted with my lack of cooperation, he staggered to his recliner and fell asleep. I called the hospice nurse to come back. When she arrived and woke up Dave, he surprised both the nurse and me. He smiled, happy to see her. He did not remember her earlier visit, nor did he remember falling, nor anything that happened after he hit his head on the cellar floor. He certainly did not know what the heck C.O. represented. He smiled at the nurse and shook his head at me. A glance of conspiracy flashed between them. I could almost read his mind.

My wife, she sure gets funny notions sometimes. C.O.? What's that?

The nurse's glance seemed sympathetic.

"He seems fine now. Keep an eye on him and call me if anything else happens."

But Dave wasn't fine. After that fall, his periods of confusion escalated. He complained of bad headaches and fell asleep in the blink of an eye. All he had to do was take one long blink and he was off to dreamland. Another result of this bad fall, Dave could no longer do his word search puzzles. He sat at table, stared down at the page, and nodded off repeatedly.

By Christmas, his appetite finally returned, but his sleepiness grew worst.

CHAPTER 42

My Best Christmas Gift

That Christmas seemed unusually quiet for Dave and me. No company expected this year, not even his sister Betty the nun who often joined us to celebrate holidays. I welcomed the day off, no big meal to fuss over. Dave didn't enjoy many foods those last weeks of his life. I planned a simple meal of chicken and rice, something he would still eat with relish. That morning, I found him in his recliner where he had slept overnight. The smell of fresh perked coffee woke him up and he came to the table without coaxing.

I knew he did not plan to attend Mass that day. Usually, if he wanted to go to church, he insisted on "cleaning up" the night before. This meant two hours in the bathroom, time enough for a chair bath, plus shaving his face. He had problems shaving now. His fingers tingled, numb with neuropathy, so he could not hang on to the razor without fumbling it away. We installed little rubber hand-holds around the shank, but even that extra thickness did little to help his shaky grip. An electric razor sat unused. He hated the way it pinched the creases in his face. The last time he tried to shave, he came out of the bathroom with his face so cut up, it looked as if it had been butchered with a dull axe.

Christmas morning he sat at the table enjoying homemade bread and butter dunked into fresh coffee. I dressed for church, then risked a quick dog walk before I left for Mass. I returned, out of breath from the cold air and the exertion of shoveling icy snow off the deck. I shrugged off my heavy coat and took off my boots before I entered the kitchen.

Dave lay face down on the kitchen table. Heart in my throat, I shook him.

Surely God, you won't take him on Christmas?

Dave's head jerked up. He turned to look in my direction.

"I can't see!" he said.

Dave wore a slice of buttered bread stuck to his glasses.

Laughter bubbled up in my throat. Giggling hysterically, I peeled his glasses off his ears and went to the sink to wash them. My shoulders shook as I removed the bread and butter and handed it to the dog. Smokey loved homemade bread and butter too. He enjoyed the unexpected treat. Both Dave and I thoroughly enjoyed the best laugh we had shared in months.

"This is the best Christmas present you have ever given me, Dave."

*Thank you, God, for reminding me that even during
the darkest days, you share your sense of humor
with your beloved children.*

CHAPTER 43

January

New Year's day we had a wonderful family gathering. Rose and her family came down and thankfully, Flo acted as chef. The house seemed blessedly full with Rose and Flo, grandson Larry, his wife Nicki and baby boy, Jesse, plus granddaughter Anna, and her daughter, Sierra. Sister Betty and brother John rounded out the table full of family members. We had stuffed shells, and several side dishes, plus three different pies. Dave ate well, if silently, and lingered long at the table, enjoying the multitude of delicious food. He managed to stay awake until the dishes were done and everyone moved to the living room. Soon his attention faded and so did he, falling asleep in his chair.

Company left around seven. They all had a long journey home. The house seemed too quiet then. Dave sound asleep, dog snoring in his bed, me watching something boring on television. I went to bed early. Dave refused to stir from his chair, so I covered him with a second blanket and let him sleep. It was past midnight when he woke me up, in a panic. He leaned over my pillow, gasping for breath.

"I'm cold!" he said, but he refused to get into bed so I could warm him up.

I heard him stumbling around in the bathroom, muttering and groaning, hangers hitting the floor of our walk-in closet. When I opened the connecting door, I found him in the closet. He was fingering his shirts, a confused and frightened expression wrinkling his face.

"I don't have any warm clothes to wear!"

Hugging him with an extra blanket, I coaxed him back to bed, shoes and all. I grabbed up more blankets and piled them on top, trying to quell his shivering panic. As he grew calmer, I risked going to the refrigerator to grab up some medicine the nurse left for "emergencies." Haldol, a sedative.

"Here, Dave. The nurse said you should take this now. It will help you."

He accepted the small spoonful and shook his head at the bitter taste. It took fifteen minutes to calm him, but his panting and groaning finally grew quiet and his breathing slowed down. I climbed into bed beside him and wrapped him in my arms. Finally, he dozed off into a fitful sleep at 2:30 a.m. Scary night.

The following days I noticed he was definitely slowing down. He forgot many of his usual routines. He never knew what time it was or where he previously sat at our table. We had maintained a routine seating arrangement for the twenty years we lived here. Dave sat to my left and no family member ever dared to sit in Dad's chair. When we recovered the kitchen chairs, I insisted we put some clear plastic on Dad's chair to protect the new material from his frequent spills. His shaky hands resulted in many dropped food items and splashed liquids. Suddenly, Dave refused to sit in his usual chair. Maybe he resented the plastic cover? I never asked why, but now he sat in a different chair at any meal he attended. Just getting him to come to the table was struggle enough. I did not have the energy to insist he sit at "Dad's place" anymore.

He often wandered through the house like a man lost in time and space. The Hospice doctor came for a visit. He agreed that Dave was definitely altered. The fact that Dave barely spoke anymore meant he was drifting away into some private world of his own. So sad to see this decline. He often refused to take his medication, despite the many times I explained their purpose. Several times I would pick up his pain pill and explain slowly.

"This is for your pain, Dave. If you only take one pill, this is the one to take!"

Sometimes he would take it routinely, other times he turned away, his eyes hooded and suspicious. I needed to reassure him continually.

"Dave, I am your wife, not your enemy. Believe me, I am only trying to help you."

Sadly he no longer believed me.

January 7th. Dave shook me awake at 2:00 a.m. "I need help!"

He had been wandering all over the main floor. Every light was turned on, even a small bulb hidden in a bookcase. He was searching for, "Something I lost." It took me a long time to get him back to bed. He kept insisting, "I need help."

It took two doses of Haldol to calm him. I hugged him as he dozed beside me. Two hours later, he lurched to his feet and went into the bathroom. Later, at the breakfast table, he still acted pretty confused. He did eat a bowl of cereal, before heading to his recliner for a long nap. Meanwhile I called Hospice and two workers came, both his nurse and my social worker.

Previously I had scheduled an oil change for the car, but had to move the date to the following week. Dave's mental state had declined to the point where I could no longer leave him alone. We were running out of daily food, so I asked friends to pick up some essentials, milk, eggs, bread.

Thank you, God, for good friends and neighbors.

A hospice volunteer, Steve, came at my request and installed a lock on the basement door. I had awakened one night to find the door wide open and the lights turned on. I did not want to find my husband lying dead at the foot of those steps. Steve also offered to stay with Dave next week so I could take the car into the dealer and pick up some food.

Dave seemed so slow moving and confused those days. He continued to fight taking his medications, including the sedatives. Hospice called this phase of Alzheimer's disease *sun-downing*. He had his days and nights mixed up. Sleep all day, roam the house all night.

One evening, he came to bed, lay down beside me. Then immediately got up and dressed himself again. I found him in the kitchen just after midnight. He stood at one end of our kitchen table, leaning on his hands and staring down at the four familiar place mats.

"Nice set-up these guys have here," he said sarcastically.

I wondered what guys he meant? His confusion seemed so sad to me. What fear-filled thoughts kept him so upset and worried that he couldn't relax into sleep? It took a good bit of persuasion but I finally got him back in bed. As I "spooned" around him, his body shook with strong tremors. His body jerked awake again and again as he struggled to relax into sleep. At 3:00 a.m., he flung the covers back and got up.

Because I felt sick myself, sharp pains in my stomach from a brewing case of food poisoning, I remained in bed, too exhausted to follow him around the house. When I dragged myself out of bed shortly after 5:00 a.m., I found him leaning on the table again. He had dressed himself in underwear and shoes. The vacuum cleaner in the closet was knocked over and rugs kicked around in the bathroom. It took a bit of struggle but I managed to button a flannel shirt around him, but he refused to wear jeans.

"I'm thirsty."

He refused to sit down as I handed him a glass of water. Of

course, his shaky hands spilled it all over the tablecloth. I cleaned that up and turned away.

"Dave, I don't have the strength to baby you right now. My belly is killing me."

I ignored his angry expression and headed for my recliner.

God! Please help me!

Using an old hangover remedy, I sipped flat cola and nibbled on crackers, trying to quiet my stomach pains and quell the nausea. It seemed too early in the morning to call Hospice so I waited. Meanwhile, Dave sat at the table to eat his breakfast, cereal with milk. When I checked later, I found him spooning cereal and milk into the case containing his hearing aids.

"Dave! Really?"

He must have recognized the reproach in my voice because he consented to put on his jeans with my help. Once dressed again, he stood up and refused to sit down. I ignored his childish behavior which seemed to work better than nagging or coaxing. He stood, weaving from side to side in the kitchen for a long time. I sat in the living room, clutching my sore belly and trying not to puke. Finally, he headed toward his recliner. He took two steps without using his cane and fell over the dog. Smokey yelped and Dave cussed. I closed my eyes and prayed. When I opened them a moment later, Dave had made his way to his recliner on hands and knees, pulled himself up and sat back. Soon he was snoring.

Hospice nurse came and went. She again offered to put Dave in "respite care," which meant Dave would go to a nursing home while I rested. Tempting, but I knew once Dave was committed to a nursing home, he would go downhill quickly. He hated hospitals. So we struggled on for a few more days.

January 13th. Nurse came early. She told me not to insist Dave take his medications. Steve the hospice worker agreed to take my car in for its oil change. The Sheriff came to replace Dave's GPS bracelet, which he had cut off the day before. He flatly refused to wear the new one. Even with those two fully armed lawmen looming over him, Dave stood his ground. He would not wear that bracelet again. Period. The Sheriff glanced at me. I shrugged.

"He doesn't go outside anymore. He can barely walk two steps without falling down."

Dave bristled at my words, thinking I was putting him down, but I spoke truth. The men nodded, their glances reflected sympathy. They left after politely offering a handshake to Dave. He turned away, his eyes suspicious.

That afternoon, while waiting for a kind neighbor to deliver some much-needed food items, Dave tried a new stunt. Standing near his recliner, he stiffened his body and fell backwards. I reached for him, trying to catch him before he hit the floor yet another time. He grabbed my shirt and we fell together in a tangled heap. We banged heads, hard. I saw stars. Rubbing my forehead, I burst into tears.

O God, this is just too much! I can't be strong anymore for Dave or for You. Please help me!

Dave stared at me as I cried on and on. Crying is unusual for me. After years of practice, I can stem any tears that spring into my eyes by swallowing hard and turning away. But this deliberate attack on me (as I saw it at the time) by the husband I had loved for so many years seemed the ultimate betrayal.

"Why?" I said, wailing. "Why do you do these hurtful things to me? I am your *wife, not your enemy!*"

I couldn't stop crying, swiping at my face like a heartbroken child.

"You hurt me, Dave!"

Finally a glimmer of the real Dave gleamed in his eyes. He reached for me, patted my back and stroked my face.

"I'm sorry," he said.

Dave never realized how much those words meant to me at that moment, and now, years later. Because, after we climbed painfully to our feet, he performed the same stunt. He stiffened his body and fell back into his recliner. It was not a fall, but a deliberate trick. In his childish state, he might have thought it was fun. Only God knows what Dave was thinking those last days of his illness.

January 14th. Rose came that night for a surprise visit. She only stayed for a few hours, but she wanted to see her father again. After supper, Dave became upset. He roamed the house searching for something important. The harder he searched, the more upset he became. Finally he told me what he *needed, right now.* He had misplaced his chewing tobacco. After a long futile search of both house and garage, we all came up empty. Dave paced the house, waving his hands, very agitated.

"Rose, I hate to ask you, but could you drive to Leeper and buy Dad his tobacco?"

She rushed out the door. When she returned with two containers, she handed them to her father. He grabbed them and shoved them into his pocket.

"Aren't you going to thank Rose for buying your stuff?"

He stared at the floor like a naughty kid and refused to answer. I noticed the hurt in her eyes when he ignored my plea that he hug her goodbye. Dad was famous for his enthusiastic hugs. Now his arms hung down as Rose stepped closer to him. He did not push her away, *thank God*, as she hugged him. Neither did he respond.

"Bye Dad. I love you."

Sad to admit, but the "real Dad" was gone now.

January 15th, Woke up that morning after a restless night in my recliner. Dave had stayed awake all night long, pacing the floor and getting into mischief while I slept. I found water in the kitchen sink. The two containers of tobacco that Rose had so kindly bought for him were floating in several inches of cold water. *So much for gratitude,* I thought bitterly as I remembered Rose's hasty trip to the store the night before. When I opened the drawer to grab silverware for breakfast, the tray was filled with water, too. Spoons were floating. All this water play from a man whose avowed enemy had been cold water in any shape or form.

Remembering Dave's rejection of cereal the day before, I tried making him eggs for his morning meal. He almost smiled as I placed the plate of two fried eggs, sunny side up, soft yolks, in front of him. He sat in a chair near the napkin holder. As I sliced bread so he could dip it in his eggs, I noticed he had taken paper napkins and was using them to dip in the yolks. I slid the napkins away and replaced them with bread. While he was occupied, I used the bathroom.

My food poisoning (from a jar of home canned peaches) seemed even worse this morning, plus I had a new symptom, pain while voiding. I groaned. Great! Another urinary track infection. A wave of helplessness washed over me.

O God, please help me. I am too sick to take care of Dave. I can't keep him safe anymore. Please hear my prayer and send me help!

I returned to my recliner and sat, helpless, as Dave staggered around the living room. He refused to use his cane. Shaky and unsteady on his feet, every few steps he fell down. Take two steps. Fall down. Cuss. Roll over, climb to his feet. Stand, weaving a bit as he regained his balance, then venture a few steps. Fall down. Cuss. Roll over.

I watched, wincing every time his body hit the floor. He ignored my pleas to sit down or to use his cane for balance. No. He acted like the two-year-old child he had become, the rebellious toddler determined to have his own way regardless of how many times he hit the floor. After a while he began to feel his way around the room, using furniture for balance. On one trip around, he noticed the long handled broom I used to sweep the front porch. Its blue handle leaned against the end of the television stand. Dave examined it for long moments, then put the end into his mouth. He blew into it, and grinned like a happy baby. Moving on, he fell heavily again, near his recliner. I hoped he would sit down finally, but he moved on. The next trip around the living room, he grabbed the blue handle and sucked on it.

Next he felt his way into the kitchen. I heard the click-click of a gas igniter on my stove. Too weak to jump to my feet, I yelled loudly.

"Leave my stove alone! That is *my* stove. Keep away from it!"

His reply sounded exactly like the child he had morphed into, "*OK!*"

I called Hospice for help. My strength gone, I was ready to give up. I could no longer keep Dave safe at home.

God, help him, now. I just can't do this any longer.

Nursing Home Blues

Two nurses came to the house within an hour. They took one look at me, so pale and weak unable to climb from my recliner, and ordered an ambulance, *for me!*

Traitor body! In the emergency room, they ordered blood work, and other tests, including a cat scan of my stomach. I lay on my side trying not to weep as the nurses and doctors fussed over me. I did not belong in the hospital. I needed to be home, taking care of Dave. But as usual, when I believe I should be in charge of my life, God steps in and takes over.

Thank you, God.

When they released me, a kindly neighbor picked me up and drove me home. As I walked in the front door, Dave sat sleeping at the kitchen table, with the two nurses watching him. They put fingers to their lips, a signal to be quiet. I snuck into the bedroom and climbed under the covers. I had given up. Betrayed by my weakened body, I covered my head and wept.

Later, the wheelchair van finally arrived to take Dave to the nursing home. I heard the nurses talking and joking with Dave as they coaxed him down the ramp and into the van.

"Look at this nice sunny day, Dave. Let's go for a ride!"

His childishly cheerful voice echoed behind him.

"Go for a ride!"

It was the last coherent speech I ever heard from my husband of 62 years.

The nurses told me later that Dave, upon his arrival at the nursing facility voiced his disapproval in no uncertain terms.

"GET ME OUT OF HERE!"

Advised by hospice nurses and the staff of the nursing home, I stayed home for several days. They told me Dave needed time to adjust to his new surroundings. So, from Thursday, the 15th, to Sunday, January 18th, I stayed home, took my medication, and rested.

That Sunday, Sister Betty came to visit. We went to Mass together, and then drove up to the nursing home to visit Dave. We arrived at lunch time. In the communal dining room, an aide sat spooning food into Dave's mouth. As soon as we sat down next to Dave's wheelchair, he clammed up and refused any further food. I emptied my pocket of the mini-candy bars he loved and scattered them across the table. He wouldn't even look at them or at me, but turned his head away and stared blankly at the wall.

Sister Betty touched his arm and spoke to him. No response. Soon his head drooped and hung down. He studied his lap until he fell asleep. A week later, Rose came to visit him but he would not meet her eyes either. By this time, he no longer sat upright in his wheelchair, but folded his body forward until his nose touched his knees. Oldest daughter Cathy could not rouse him either when she visited that weekend. Our oldest grandsons, Dave III and Chris also visited their grandpa with the same results. He had been put into bed at my request after I saw him bent over in his chair, and noticed the other patients avoiding him as if his illness was catching.

The staff called me with updates every day.

"Dave won't take his medication anymore."

"Dave stopped accepting food. An aide had to remove food from his mouth this morning because he refused to swallow it."

Dave's life was ebbing away and it was killing me with guilt.

God! Dave should be here, at home with me. Not stuck in a nursing home with strangers who don't love him or take care of him with love and affection, the way I would.

Except I couldn't take care of him anymore. And the thought of my inadequacies haunted my restless sleep.

January 26th. That Monday, I took a chance on the winter weather and went to town to stock up on food. My fridge and cupboards were empty. Smokey needed dog food too. It had snowed a lot that weekend but the main roads were clear. Not my driveway. I almost got stuck coming home, sliding toward the ditch as my faithful 4-wheel drive car spun up the driveway. Usually my niece, who lived in the original homestead just below our house, had her husband, Dan, plow us out. I had mentioned it twice on social media that my driveway needed a plow. But she failed to see my message asking for help. That Monday, after struggling to get into the garage, then putting away the groceries, I collapsed into deep depression, fueled by the unplowed driveway. The next day, the latest message from the staff at the nursing home made me frantic.

"Mrs. Bauer. Dave has been skipping breaths. He stops breathing an average of sixteen times a minute. You better come soon before it's too late."

I panicked. Weeping helplessly, I called Randy. This is the nephew who had always helped us. He built our ramp and did various other jobs as Dave's strength faded with age.

Randy listened patiently to my hysterical tale of woe, and suggested another local man, a distant relative, who did snow plowing during the winter. Eric Bauer came within the hour and plowed me out both front and back. His only fee? A warm hug of thanksgiving.

Thanks God, for loving people
willing to help out in an emergency.

CHAPTER 45

The Final Hours

Tuesday, January 27th. Dave lay flat on his back in his bed, his mouth hanging open. His eyes were dark as he stared sightlessly at nothing. I had come after lunch, with a bag full of snacks and water for me, fortification for a long vigil at Dave's bedside. I sat down beside his bed and took his limp hand. His eyes flickered briefly, but did not focus on me. We sat there for long hours. Me holding his hand, he struggling to breathe through his open mouth.

Dave's brother John and his wife Patty came and stayed for a while. They left as winter twilight approached. I sat and prayed. The nurses were extra kind. They even brought me a tray for supper. The aides came and turned Dave on his other side, after changing his diaper and washing his body. I moved to the recliner against the wall. After a long time, I thought to call my kind neighbor, Sue. Her daughter brought her up to stay with me. Sue's husband, Wish, had died the previous year. How much courage it must have taken for her to join me in the deathwatch of my husband, when she had lost her beloved just a short year before!

We sat and talked quietly. At one point, I noticed Dave's expression had changed. I stood up to stare at his face. *He was smiling!* His lips were wide open as he grinned from ear to ear. I had never seen him so happy, never. He stared at something above the bed. His lips were stretched so wide I could see his gums.

Sue said quietly, "He must be seeing somebody he loves."

I sank back in the recliner as Dave's smile faded.

"I wonder who he sees? Jim, maybe? Or his mother?"

"Probably Jesus, you think, Cecile?"

I nodded, overwhelmed with gratitude for that special smile on the face of my dying husband.

Thank you, God, for that brief glimpse of heavenly happiness. I know Dave will be home with you soon. Strengthen me with the courage to let him go, O God of all eternity.

Sue and I stayed awake, watching, as Dave quietly slept. He was on oxygen now, and it seemed to help him. At 3 a.m. I stood up and put my finger on a pulse in his neck.

"Nice and strong, Sue. I think his heart will keep him going for a while yet. Maybe we should go home and get some rest?"

We were both exhausted. I worried about Sue as the long vigil dragged on. She suffered heart problems, and I did not want her to have another attack. I knew keeping her with me meant she had to relive her own painful deathbed vigil of last year. I got up and reached for my cane.

Sue stood up too. "You sure?"

I nodded. "He has a way to go, yet. We both need some rest."

I glanced back at Dave as we headed toward the door. His eyes seemed full of reproach as we walked away. I thought of Jesus in the Garden of Gethsemane.

Could you not watch with me for one hour?

But we did need to rest. I kissed Dave and patted his hand.

"See you tomorrow, Hon."

All the way home I fought the urge to return to Dave. I hated to leave him there alone.

What if? What if he died during the night? Please, God, keep him safe in your care.

The next morning, he was still breathing, still alive, still waiting for me.

CHAPTER 46

But Nobody Came

Caught too few hours of sleep that night/morning, made a few necessary phone calls, and then headed back to the nursing home. It was just past 9:00 a.m. when I walked into his room. A privacy curtain screened his bed from the doorway. I pushed it aside.

"Good morning, Sweetheart," I said as I kissed his forehead.

His eyes were open. Did I see a flicker of recognition in their dark depths? I leaned closer to whisper.

"It's OK to let go now, Dave. God and our boys are waiting for you. The kids are coming. I'll be all right. Go with God, Honey."

No answering flicker, but he did heave a long sigh. I kissed him again before moving to the recliner. Arranging my purse, cane, and water bottle on the nearby window sill, I settled in for another long day. Folding my hands, I finished the Rosary prayer. Every morning, while walking the dog, I began that ancient comforting prayer given to the people of earth by Jesus' mother, Mary. In my rush to return to Dave, it had been a short dog walk that day. Not enough time to pray all five decades. As I counted off the beads, I prayed fervently that Dave would not suffer pain that day as his body slowly shut down.

It seemed extra quiet in his room that sunny morning. Dave breathed in, breathed out. Occasionally, he coughed. I watched his chest rise and fall. Breathe in, breathe out. No one entered the room to check on Dave at all. The night before, every fifteen minutes a nurse, doctor, or aide would come in to see Dave. Not this morning.

Breathe in. Breathe out.

And then he stopped. He took one final breath, closed his eyes, and died.

I sat up straighter and stared at him. No more breathing. His chest did not move again.

I leaped to my feet to stare down at him. He looked peaceful, relaxed. No more struggle to breathe. No more coughing.

No more pain, no more struggles. He is with Me now. He is at peace in My Kingdom.

The whisper in my mind had to be from the One who loves us beyond the grave. I kissed my husband and said my final goodbye with tears and prayers.

I glanced at the wall clock. Dave died at 10:20 a.m. on Wednesday, January 28.

Sniffling into a handkerchief, I pushed the nurse's call button, and sat down to wait.

But nobody came.

I cried more tears. Glanced at the clock. Five minutes had passed. Still nobody came. I stood up on shaky legs and reached for the call button. Maybe I hadn't pushed it hard enough?

Ten minutes later, still no one entered Dave's death room.

Nobody came.

Muttering to myself, I grabbed my cane and stomped down the long hallway to the nurses' station. A group of laughing people huddled around the counter. No one glanced my way for long moments. I felt tempted to throw my cane at someone to catch their attention. Finally one woman looked up. Her smiling face changed as she stared at me. I was so angry and upset I couldn't even talk. I gestured back at the hallway, shook my head, and gave her a thumbs down. I turned and stomped back. Before I had stumbled four steps, the doctor passed me as she raced toward Dave's room. I found her bent over Dave's still form, listening to his chest with her stethoscope. She looked up at me and shook her head.

"I'm sorry, Mrs. Bauer, but he's gone."

"I knew that fifteen minutes ago! He died at 10:20. I rang for the nurse, but nobody came!"

She wanted to list the time of death as 10:35 a.m., the time she finally came to the room to pronounce him dead. When I insisted she write down the actual time he stopped breathing, she backed off a bit.

"Let's split the difference, shall we? I'll write time of death at 10:25 a.m."

Suddenly all my strength left me. What did it matter what numbers appeared on a chart? Dave, my sweetheart for over sixty years, was gone. That terrible knowledge sucked all the strength from my body. I collapsed into the recliner, too exhausted to even argue anymore.

I did have enough presence of mind to ask the doctor to call Borland's Funeral Home.

"Greg is waiting for your call," I said. "I talked to him this morning"

I sat at the foot of the bed and watched as two aides washed and shaved Dave. I marveled at their matter-of-fact efficiency. As they washed his lower body, I noticed just how thin he had become. His legs were skinny enough to belong to a ten year old kid, not a man in his eighties. Lividity streaks already marked his back. After death, blood pools in the lowest body parts. It had been less than a half-hour since my honey died, and already the early signs of decomposition were present. I sat and watched, too numb to really take it all in, as the aides prepared Dave's body for the mortician.

Greg arrived with a gurney and his helper. I had waited to talk to him about the funeral arrangements. He hugged me first and expressed his sincere sympathy.

"Greg, can you hold off on the obituary for a day? I need to talk to the West Coast kids. I know they will come, but nobody knows their flight plans yet."

He agreed, as he skillfully attended to my honey. With quiet dignity, he slid Dave into a black body bag, and then transferred him onto the gurney. His glance filled me with quiet comfort.

"Is there anything else I can do for you, now?"

I shook my head and picked up my purse. He touched my arm.

"Is it all right if I stop by later this afternoon? We'll need to pick up his clothing, and some photographs for the computer screen display we use at Wakes."

I nodded. It would take me all afternoon to go through the old pictures, but by the time Greg came out to the house, I had everything ready. As I handed him Dave's good suit, shirt and tie, I also included a surprise. Sister Betty had given her brother a pair of red/white/blue suspenders a couple of years before. Dave wore them once, to please his older sibling, but really, they were too flashy for Dave's taste. He had always been a modest man, in dress and behavior.

I explained the suspenders and grinned.

"Dave wouldn't wear these. But I always loved them and I want him to wear them now."

"Uh oh, asking for trouble, Cecile," Greg said and grinned. "Dave might find a way to get even with you. The newly dead have a way of getting their payback, even from heaven."

I laughed at the thought, but Greg's warning proved to be accurate. Dave got even for those suspenders, big time.

CHAPTER 47

The Final Goodbye

I spent the rest of that day making and receiving telephone calls from friends and relatives. Sister Betty offered to come down from Pittsburgh the next day, but I put her off.

"Thanks, Sister, but I need a day to myself. To rest, to gather my wits, to pray. I hope you understand."

She did, thank God, so I had one free day before the house filled up with family. I used that day to knead what I called "Rosary Bread." I called it that because I recited a decade of the Rosary as I kneaded up the dough. The familiar prayer seemed to make the dough extra smooth, which resulted in especially delicious loaves. The fifty-year-old recipe made a dozen loaves of homemade white bread. Family was coming! They were all raised on this homemade bread. Dave loved it too. As I formed the pliant dough into loaves, I remembered how, in his last days, Dave had eaten nothing but bread and butter. No other food tempted him then. It was my homemade bread and butter or nothing.

My children began arriving the next day. Tom came first, late on that Friday evening. He rented a car from the airport in Pittsburgh and drove through a snowstorm for three hours before coming up my now completely plowed driveway. My niece's husband had been faithful at keeping the area clear of snow ever since that terrible Tuesday when another relative had plowed me out. I had straightened up the second bay of the garage so Tom could park his rental inside. That garage door opener sometimes gave me trouble and that night was no exception. It would go down, then hesitate at the bottom and go back up again. Tom and I worked together for long cold minutes before we finally got the door to stay down. I ended up standing on the bottom handle and swearing at it before it yielded and stayed in the down position.

"Is Dad playing tricks on us, Mom?"

I had to laugh.

"Could be, Tom. You never know what your father might do."

Jason from Arizona, plus Barb and her Henry, Jean and her youngest son, Nate, all from northern California arrived next. As they usually did when visiting here, this group of West Coast adult children coordinated their flights and shared a rented van. Rose and her family came down too. Later Cathy and Mike arrived and stayed overnight.

It felt so good to have the house full of family again! They dove into the homemade bread and jam like starving cats. Lots of chatter, some tears, but laughter too, as they hugged and retold the old stories. Siblings conferred and made beer runs. We all relaxed as the family settled into what all of them considered their second, and (often) summer vacation home. The beds upstairs filled up fast. Some slept on sleeping bags or in the living room recliners. Other family members made reservations at local motels. The house was full and I felt safe and contented, surrounded by the people I love best, my adult children and grandchildren.

Donated food filled up both refrigerators and all the counters. In this rural area of Pennsylvania, whenever a family suffers a death, neighbors, relatives and friends head for their kitchens to whip up food for "mourners." Food and more food. Lots of desserts, main dishes, lunch meat, rolls, whatever could be made quickly and delivered to our door, appeared as if magic, and was just as quickly devoured with relish by our hungry hoard of Bauer kin.

The first Viewing was scheduled for Sunday afternoon, March 1st. Snow fell heavily as we drove the two miles to Leeper. We carpooled, using the rented van, and other vehicles parked around the house. I didn't care who I rode with, I just refused to drive. Not that driving in snow scared me. I just wanted to relax before the trauma of the funeral home and its stressful routine. Dave had a good crowd for his Viewing that afternoon. Our pastor, Father Christopher, came before the official visiting hours and performed the Vigil service for the family. We arrived early to have this private time to grieve before friends and other relatives started coming.

The family walked slowly past the coffin, most cried, others stared off, blinking back good memories of their father and grandfather. Most echoed a familiar refrain.

Dad looks good. Peaceful. No more pain on his face.

I pulled Sister Betty closer to the coffin and showed her Dave's suspenders. She backed away, as if afraid to touch or get so personal with her deceased brother. A surprise to me. I thought nuns had a different mind-set about dead people. I knew the body in the coffin was just the earthly shell of the real Dave. My husband had escaped this veil of tears and lived on, in spirit, safe with our heavenly Father.

People came, gave hugs and sincere expressions of sympathy. Time passed in a blur. My arms ached from hugging everyone. I sat down frequently to rest my painful knee. Before we knew it, time had passed and the first Viewing was over. Snow fell steadily as we headed home. Jay drove the rented van up the long hill leading to our house. He bit his lips as the tires spun and the vehicle wandered toward the ditch. He had been a desert dweller for too many years. No snow in Arizona, I guess.

"Just keep the wheels straight, Jay. They're not whining yet. You'll get up this hill all right. Just keep your foot steady and the wheels straight."

He listened to my advice. Sure enough we topped the hill, cheered on by the back seat riders, and got home safely. People laughed as they piled out of the van.

"Thought we might have to push you out, Jay."

"Yeah, yeah!"

After an extravagant supper, provided by our generous friends and neighbors, we shrugged into coats for the evening Viewing. A quick discussion led to me handing the keys to my SUV to Jason.

"It has 4-wheel drive, Jay. You can drive through anything in it."

We left the van parked behind the house.

As the evening Viewing dragged by, I kept watching the windows. Snow, heavy snow, fell outside. Greg Borland spent most of the evening shoveling off the sidewalks that led to the funeral home doors. No new visitors arrived. By 7:30 p.m., I made a decision. Gathering the family, I canceled the rest of the Wake.

"I don't think anybody else will come in this blizzard. We might as well go home."

They all nodded and raced for their coats. Greg met us at the door, shovel in hand. He grinned at me.

"Told you Dave would get even with you about those suspenders, Cecile."

"Yep," I said and had to smile. "Dave really did hate those garish suspenders."

Grandson Larry, his wife, Nicki, and their baby Jesse stayed behind, just in case someone braved the bad winter weather to attend the last half hour of Dave's Wake. The rest of us waded through the parking lot, swept off the cars, and headed home. My car had no problem climbing the hill, but other people didn't make it. Several adult grandchildren ended up backing down the hill and heading, instead, to town and their rented rooms. But the majority of our family got home safely. We stomped into the house, grateful for good tires and 4-wheel drive vehicles.

It was Super Bowl Sunday. When we walked into the house, football fans glanced at the clock. It was half-time. Someone asked me if I minded them watching the game.

"No, go ahead," I said and sat down in the kitchen.

Dave and I had never been football fans. Most of our adult children and grandchildren, however, were avid fans. It didn't bother me if they wanted to watch football's game of the year. Who cared? Not me. I didn't even know what teams were playing. I relaxed in the kitchen, drinking a rare beer to numb myself from thinking too much. Out in the living room, voices cheered or groaned, whenever something exciting happened. Bottles clinked. Bags of chips rattled. Someone hurried into the kitchen to fetch little bowls of chip-dip. A long groan.

"Ohhhh! There goes the ball game!"

"What a stupid play! Is the coach nuts?"

I glanced around the kitchen at the chips, dip, and empty bottles of beer. I stifled a laugh.

Dave? Can you believe this? We're hosting a Super Bowl party! And neither of us knows a thing about football.

I went to bed early.

✳✳✳

Tomorrow would be a busy day, a day to say a final goodbye to my sweet farm-boy, whom I had loved for sixty-four years. Our adult children and grandchildren would weep for the loss of the man who gave the world's best hugs. The funeral Mass would be unforgettably awesome. Our former pastor, Father Tom Hoderny, a wonderful boss both Dave and I had worked for while he was assigned to St. Mary Church, would co-celebrate the Mass. His loving tribute to Dave brought many of us to tears.

Our family served at Mass in many ways that day. Both Nicki and Andrea (Jim's widow), whose voices blended sweetly, acted as cantors as we all sang the beautiful funeral hymns. Great-grandson, four-month-old Jesse, added his cheerful voice to the singing. Grandsons Larry and Jonathan brought up the gifts. Sister Betty acted as Lector, reading the familiar passages from the Old Testament. Grandson Bryan acted as altar server, a role he had performed for the Eden church since he was in third grade there. His profound bow just before Communion made his glasses slide off his nose and provided a bit of comic relief to our aching sorrow. The Funeral liturgy was comforting, the readings and hymns sorrowfully beautiful. As the Pallbearers (grandsons and nephew, Randy) wheeled Dave's coffin down the aisle for the closing prayers, we all wept for our loss and heaven's gain.

A bitter cold snow and wind met us at the back door of the church. No one was expected to follow the coffin into the cemetery. Too much snow to walk through the deep drifts. Plus I couldn't bear to see them put my honey into the ground. We had already said our last goodbyes. After Mass, we all enjoyed a delicious funeral dinner, provided by the women of the church.

But all that would happen tomorrow.

✴✴✴

Tonight I drifted off to sleep listening to the football fans discussing the pros and cons of the game. Their voices sounded like sweet music to my ears.

Family. Home here, enjoying each other.
Thank you, God, for your multitude of blessings.
In Jesus name I pray.

Alone, Yet Not Alone

It has been over a year since my husband Dave died. I have learned so much during that time.

First and most important, I learned to rely on the Holy Spirit to guide me each day. Alone, I can do nothing. With God, all things are possible, even for a new widow, struggling to just get by in my suddenly empty house. I learned how to replace my bitterness and anger at the multitude of loved ones God had claimed. My profound grief faded as I listened to the nudging of the Holy Spirit.

Your family members are all together in a much better place. Their pain and sufferings are over now. They are happy and safe in heaven. God understands your losses. He is here to comfort you, every moment of every day. Turn to God with your tears. And he will comfort you.

After a year of bitter grief and mourning, I am on my way to peaceful acceptance. Writing this book helped immensely to sort out my raw emotions and work through my profound sorrow. At last I can weep freely for my loved ones who are safe in God's loving embrace. It is such a comfort to know my three sons and their father are all together again happy and peaceful in the eternal Kingdom.

I also learned practical things. Such as how to change a florescent light fixture (after waiting weeks for promised help that never materialized). It took me almost two hours, leaning across the bathroom sink, balancing on a 2-step stool, fingers shaking from the unfamiliar danger of working with electric-

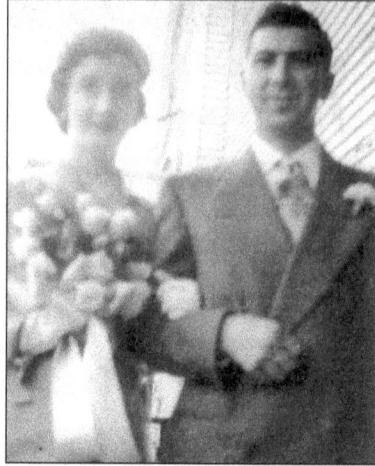

November 22, 1952, the wedding day

ity. But when that new tube light blinked on, I cheered, satisfied with my work.

I learned how to repair my favorite snow shovel. The aluminum bottom part had slid off the wooden handle. Since I didn't have another suitable shovel, and we had a really snowy winter that year, I tried to fix the old one. Working down cellar, searching through Dave's workbench for suitable tools, I dug out a tube of liquid nails. Next job, find a calking gun. Rummaging around the various items scattered across his workbench, I finally found the tool. Dave kept insisting he needed to "red up" his workbench in the weeks before his death, but of course, time caught up with his good intentions. Now I fitted the liquid nails tube into the calking gun and tried to squeeze the trigger.

No go. Hmm. Gun must be faulty.

I searched through a bucket of son Russ's tools and came up with a larger calking gun. It didn't work either. By this time, my back hurt, so I sat down and mulled over the situation. *Why isn't this working?* Finally common sense (or maybe the Holy Spirit took pity on my ignorance) solved my problem with the equipment. I needed to cut off the end of the tube before anything would squeeze out! Duh! One good squeeze

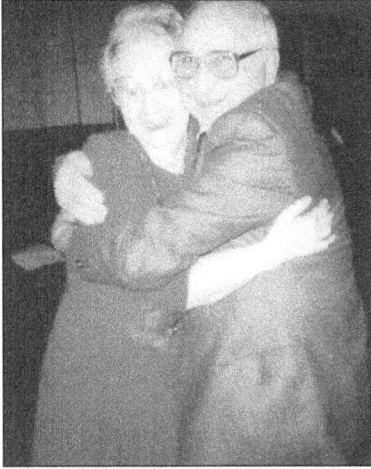

50th Anniversary Celebration in 2002

and liquid nails oozed out the end and into the slot where the shovel handle met the snow blade. While waiting for the liquid to set up, I found a short screw and installed it into a hole in the assembly. It wouldn't go all the way in, so I grabbed a hammer and forced it down with a few good whacks.

Who's your Mama? I told my adult kids, later, on social media. That shovel is still usable now, in its second winter after my repair. God takes care of widows and fools, I do believe.

That spring, I learned how to run Dave's beloved lawn mower. The riding tractor came to life, roaring loudly in the confines of the garage. It startled me. This was Dave's toy. He let me sit on it. Once. Now I needed to master it in order to cut grass. When I let out the clutch, it lurched ahead, snarling. I drove up the slanted lawn to the field at the top of our property. I figured I would start out by mowing the tall grass on my walk-path. Safer that way. Wide open field, no trees to run into. Up in the field, I noticed the cutting blades were not working. I paused and fished the manual out from under my leg and paged through it for helpful information.

"Ah, hah!"

Found the control for the cutter blades and moved it into position. With a thick vibration, grass and corn husks flew out the bottom side hopper. Yay! I was in business. By the time I finished that first excursion into the grass mowing business, I discovered why Dave's back hurt all the time. The mower rode like an old hay wagon, rattling and jostling my body back and forth. As I bounced around mowing the area around the fire ring, I thought, *This must be what hell is like: doing something I hate over rough ground.*

195

I learned how to budget my greatly reduced income. Rationed my trips to town to twice a month to save gas money. Ate less and even lost over twenty pounds, which helped reduce my knee and back pains. Made do, did without, and lived leaner. I also performed a lot of home maintenance such as painting outside, scrubbing and re-staining the front porch floor, and trimming the trees and bushes. I mastered ladder work by using stretchy straps to secure the ladder to nearby stable items, such as the porch pillars when I needed to clean leaves and debris out of the gutters. Repaired the roof on the grandkids' playhouse when wind lifted one corner of the rolled roofing. All this carpentry work reminded me of building our house, twenty years ago. I could still swing a hammer and even managed to master the power drill/screwdriver.

What helped me perform so many chores, work that I had depended on my husband to do for so many years, was making "to-do" goal lists every month. As I finished off each item, crossing it off the list gave me a sense of accomplishment.

For the first time in my long life, I had learned to live alone, despite the weirdness of a quiet house. After so many years of the hustle and bustle of daily life in a large family, now even the sound of the dog's toenails on the kitchen floor echo loudly in my ears. I am alone, but not alone. Not only do I feel the daily presence of my dearly departed family, my three sons and my husband, but the Holy Spirit whispers good words into my soul. Words that nudged me to write this family story of loving, losing and learning.

This month my goal list mentioned, "Fetch down old love letters and read them."

It took me a while to sort through those old love letters, two years of accumulated letters that Dave and I had written across the miles that separated us. We had lived in different states when we first met. I hoped to find the second letter he sent me after we met at the dance in Crown, on July 2nd, 1950. It was so sweet, that old letter, it told about all the work he performed on his father's farm. He mentioned digging coal in the family coal mine because his uncle needed a ton of coal. Price for all Dave's hard labor? $4.00. He also bragged about the good yield of wheat harvested from their acres, 93 bushels. That summer he had already begun to plow acreage for next year's crop, using two horses and a walk-behind plow. My farm-boy, at age nineteen, already did the work of a man. His letter ended on a hopeful note.

"I have to fix the barn roof this week. Hope I don't fall off, because I really want to see you again."

As I pawed through that messy pile of letters, the Holy Spirit nudged me. Out of all those disorganized envelopes, I found one marked, "special," on the outside. I turned the letter over, smiling at the upside down three cent stamp and the S.W.A.K. on the flap. Initials meant: Sealed With A Kiss. Upside down stamp meant *I love you* in that old code known well by corresponding sweethearts in the 1950's. Inside I found a letter so special that it immediately felt as if Dave had written it that day, a message straight from heaven.

Dearest, Hello darling. Here I am writing to you because I love you very much, and I am very lonely for you now. I wish you were here right now so I could take you in my arms and hug you and kiss you to show you how much I really love you sweetheart. How are you these cold winter days? (It was a cold winter's day when I re-read this very special letter.)

He signed it, *I'll always love you, Darling. Love and kisses, David Bauer.*

That signature made me grin. As if I could ever forget him or his last name. I have proudly worn that name, with the Mrs. before it, for sixty plus years: Mrs. David P. Bauer.

Love you, too, my sweet, sweet farm boy.

S. W.A. K.

Lessons Learned
Battling Alzheimer's Disease

Make no mistake, you will be fighting a formidable enemy, a disease that knows no mercy, nor gives scant hope of a happy ending, as your loved one slowly slips away. But the following tips or hints from an experienced caregiver may help make your journey easier.

1) **Pray.** Pray every day, pray all day. Pray when you feel overwhelmed. Give thanks when your loved one has a good day. Pray when you are ready to give up. Just pray! Ask for that mustard seed of hope mentioned in Matthew 17:20. But if that tiny seed of faith fails to help you, pray for something bigger: an avocado pit of patience. Worked for me!

2) **Cherish the good times,** the moments when your patient responds to you with something resembling normal good times. Laugh together. Hug your loved one. Tell him or her how much you love them. Touch them with love, as often as possible. Alzheimer's victims often feel isolated from their surroundings as memory slips away. But kisses and hugs are welcome

and appreciated, even if your spouse or parent no longer recognizes you.

3) **Sing.** If your patient is musically inclined, as many older people are, the sound of familiar songs stirs them to respond. Nurses report that even people who have not spoken in weeks, will sing Christmas songs when they hear them performed. Sadly, my husband did not appreciate music, so this remedy for his frequent depression could not help him.

4) **Child proof your house.** Alzheimer's patients gradually morph into mischievous toddlers. They will get into anything, including cleaning products stored under the sink. Pull the knobs off your stove when not cooking. If you have a basement door, install a lock and keep the key in your own pocket. Hide potent medicine in locked cabinets. Even patients who refuse their own medications, may be adventurous enough to try something new they find in a pill box on your dresser.

5) As soon as your loved one shows signs of **impaired driving** (two or more minor accidents), pull the car keys and hide them. As my husband descended into thoughtless driving habits, and despite his vigorous objections, I grounded him. He complained bitterly and criticized my own driving skills endlessly, but I could not allow him to endanger other people with

his reckless driving. Men typically equate driving with being a real man, a macho king of the road. The battle over the keys to the car may be fierce. If necessary, have your family doctor explain why he can no longer drive. The doctor's orders often carry more weight than a mere spouse!

6) **Guns and other weapons.** My loved one was a farm boy, raised on hunting for meat. We always had rifles and shotguns kept in a locked gun safe. Usually, he kept a few shells in his shotgun to ward off varmints attacking the garden. As dementia stole away his common sense, I quietly unloaded all the long guns, and hid the boxes of ammunition under skeins of yarn in my large knitting box. I also hid his car key in the same place. I kept the gun cabinet key on my key ring. My pocket held enough keys to tilt me sideways.

7) **Keys.** As mentioned above, caregivers of Alzheimer's patients needs to keep keys in their pockets. Keys to the locked doors in the house, including the doors to the outside. Keys to the car, of course, in case you need to go for help. Many a trusting caregiver has been locked out of the house by a mischievous patient, bent on doing something forbidden. I also carried my cell phone in the other pocket of my jeans. I had important numbers on speed dial, ready for any emergency.

8) **Take time to enjoy the good times.** Keep up social ties. Visit friends, family and neighbors as long as possible. Take walks together, holding hands, like sweethearts always do. If you live in a questionable neighborhood, drive to a large Mall and join the morning walkers there. Most Malls are open early, even before their stores unlock their doors, in order to accommodate the walkers. At home, play cards and board games together. Bring out the old photo albums and VCR/DVD tapes of family parties and other special occasions. As your loved one's memory fades, find something to trigger his or her interest. Women often retain their ability to knit or crochet long into their illness. Men may enjoy puzzles of any type. My husband loved Word Finder puzzles. He kept up this hobby until two weeks before he descended into the final stages of dementia.

9) **Personal hygiene.** Be aware that cleanliness often falls by the wayside as your loved one reverts to toddler habits. Don't be fooled, as I was by son Russ's charade of wet, but unwashed hair. The nose knows. Take a sniff of your patient's hair. If it smells of oil or unwashed scalp, time to schedule bath time. Sometimes this is a battle, as it was with my stubborn hubby. Just getting him to change his clothing seemed too much of a struggle for the both of us. I learned to wait until he was sound asleep in our bed, then got up, snagged

his clothing off the bedroom chair, emptied the pockets, and buried the clothing under a load of laundry in the washer. He did like to cling to familiar shirts and jeans so I did laundry often to appease him. If you belong to Hospice, they have Bath Ladies who will come and help clean up your stubborn loved one. Unfortunately, Dave's fierce modesty prevented this very necessary help for me.

10) **Take time for yourself.** Be sensible enough to realize you need time alone to regroup your energy, to calm your rattled nerves, to rest your exhausted body. Taking care of an Alzheimer's patient quickly drains your reserve of strength, patience, and peace of mind. Ask family members, friends, or the Hospice staff for help. It is not a sign of weakness, but a life saving strategy to keep you going when the going really gets rough.

11) **Safety first.** If you have an escape artist for a patient, someone who slips out of the house and wanders away, invest in a GPS bracelet. Our local Sheriff's Department sponsored these Global Positioning System bracelets for dementia patients. They had the specialized equipment that could locate a lost person no matter how deeply hidden, even in an underground cave. Dave hated his bracelet, but he wore it anyway. The peace of mind it gave me seemed worth any price.

12) **Practical concerns.** My best financial advice, for anyone contemplating the dreadful future of a loved one with dementia, is to buy nursing home insurance. If there is a family history of Alzheimer's disease, don't wait. The sooner you purchase this insurance, the cheaper it will be. During the final stages of dementia, if you can no longer take care of your loved one, as happened to me, realize that Medicare does not cover nursing home charges. If you do not have sizable cash reserves, nursing home costs can drain your bank accounts within a month. Dave's care cost thousands of dollars for the thirteen days he resided in a local facility. If you think you can rely on Medicaid, know that if you own any property, a house or land, the state Medicaid program will attach a lien onto your home until they are reimbursed for your patient's care.

13) **Finally, a word to those caregivers struggling to keep their loved one at home until the end.** There are companies with trained people who will come to your home and stay overnight to allow you to get some sleep. I wish I had taken advantage of these programs as Dave's behavior became so radical that I could no longer keep him safe. The price of an overnight caregiver is reasonable enough that we could have managed it. Far cheaper than the nursing home costs. My husband was on the cusp of becoming bed-ridden when I gave up and allowed him to be taken away.

A few days of restful sleep was all I really needed to resume my duties. Your local doctor would be the person to ask for a reference. The Hospice nurses may also be willing to give out the information, even though the companies compete for business.

God bless you and keep you strong as you care
for your loved one, in Jesus' name I pray.

www.ingramcontent.com/pod-product-compliance
Lightning Source LLC
LaVergne TN
LVHW011347080426
835511LV00005B/175